SOUND THERAPY
MUSIC TO RECHARGE YOUR BRAIN

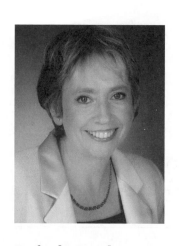

Rafaele Joudry

Born in England and educated in
Canada, Rafaele migrated to Australia in
1980, where she worked as a community
developer for six years. She then joined
her mother in launching the self-help
Sound Therapy system and established
Sound Therapy International in 1989.
She has delivered over 500 lectures
on Sound Therapy around Australia,
North America and Europe, has given
dozens of TV and Press interviews and has
authored three books on the subject. She is
committed to making Sound Therapy
available to everyone who needs it.

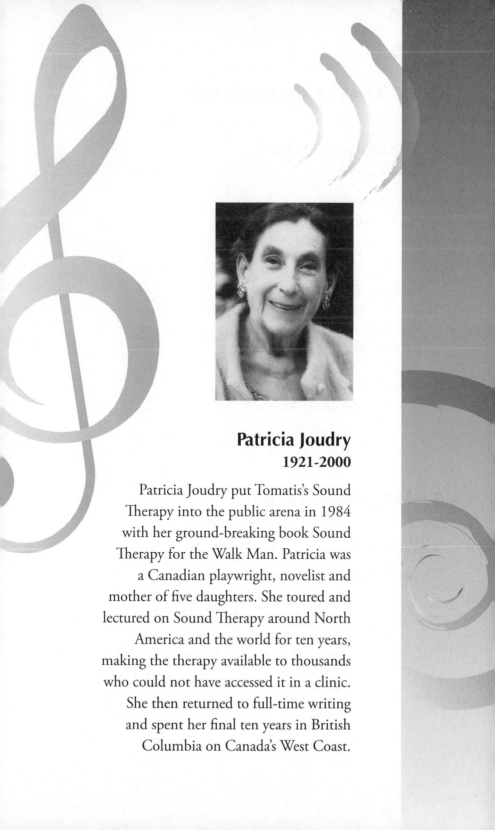

Patricia Joudry
1921-2000

Patricia Joudry put Tomatis's Sound Therapy into the public arena in 1984 with her ground-breaking book Sound Therapy for the Walk Man. Patricia was a Canadian playwright, novelist and mother of five daughters. She toured and lectured on Sound Therapy around North America and the world for ten years, making the therapy available to thousands who could not have accessed it in a clinic. She then returned to full-time writing and spent her final ten years in British Columbia on Canada's West Coast.

Other books by Patricia Joudry

Novels
The Dweller on the Threshold
The Selena Tree

Autobiography
And the Children Played
Spirit River to Angels' Roost

Plays
Teach Me How to Cry
The Song of Louise in the Morning
The Sand Castle
A Very Modest Orgy

Metaphysical
Twin Souls co-author Maurie D. Pressman M.D.

Books by Rafaele Joudry

Sound Therapy: Music to Recharge Your Brain

Triumph Over Tinnitus

Why Aren't I Learning?

SOUND THERAPY

MUSIC TO RECHARGE YOUR BRAIN

Patricia Joudry

Rafaele Joudry

A SUCCESS STREAM BOOK

First published as *Sound Therapy for the Walk Man* in 1984
  by Sound Therapy Canada.
Reprinted 1984 (twice), 1985, 1986, 1989, 1994 (twice), 1996.

Revised editions published by
  Sound Therapy International,
  2/9 Bergin St Gerringong NSW 2534
  Australia.
Revised edition entitled *Sound Therapy: Music to Recharge Your Brain*, published in 1999
  and reprinted in 2000, 2001, 2007.
This newly revised edition printed in 2009.
Reprinted 2013.

National Library of Australia Cataloguing-in-Publication entry
Author: Joudry, Patricia, 1921-2000.
Title: Sound therapy : music to recharge your brain / Patricia Joudry, Rafaele Joudry.
Edition: 12th ed.
ISBN: 9780957924642 (pbk.)
Notes: Includes index.
            Bibliography.
Subjects: Music therapy.
            Sound--Psychological aspects.
Other Authors/Contributors:
            Joudry, Rafaele.
Dewey Number:
            615.85154

'Sony' and 'Walkman' ™ are registered trademarks of Sony Corporation, Tokyo, Japan.
Typesetting: www.ePrintDesign.com.au
Cover design: Michelle Rajcany, M Design www.mdesign.net.au
Printed by C.O.S Printers, Singapore.

Contents

Foreword to the First Edition

By Yehudi Menuhin 1916–1999

  ❝ *The ear collects the spiralling energy from the cosmos, this* ❞
energy gives life to man and we see this vitality in the light
which shines forth from our eyes.

Tibetan Medical Doctor

I was fascinated by this book, which I read between dawn and breakfast at one sitting! I am prepared to believe that the therapy is a very valuable form of rehabilitation affecting more than the brain, important though that is. It also substantiates the value and use of music.

Music is the voice of the universe, it is the voice of humanity and is part of our existence. Good music is the harmonization of all the vibrations of which matter consists, and it restores us to ourselves and to our universe. It is the bond that we have between our own frequencies and those frequencies which vibrate millions of light years away.

When we hear music we are actually vibrating with the whole audience, and with the performer, and we are thereby put in touch with the composer's mind and heart.

I have always felt that music is basically therapeutic, restoring proportions which are squeezed out of shape by the pressures of the day. In a state of physical disequilibrium of the nerves or the mind, music can reach our subconscious and put things in place. And now this therapy is exploring a fascinating new approach to the inner human being. It comes at a time when we are literally being deafened by the rising noise level in our world. The decibel volume is growing with every year and is destroying our hearing and deadening us to our environment.

We seem to think that the ear is dispensable. We concentrate overwhelmingly on what is visual. Everything that we cultivate or build impresses through the eyes, by size and colour and shape. We ignore the miracle of the ear, which conveys its message through a greater abstraction than sound. Sound goes directly into our bodies. What the aural can do to the inside of our brain, to the "within" of our lives, nothing else can do.

The use of the higher vibrations, as described in this book, opens a whole new world to us. Sound Therapy has a specific effect which seems to have wide implications and to yield undreamed of results. I believe that it constitutes a breakthrough to a new level of effectiveness in music and health.

Yehudi Menuhin continued to explore his interest in the purpose of harmonies in the universe, the therapeutic applications of sound and the influence of sound on the development of the brain and the human being. Through his life he sustained a belief in advancing human consciousness and the power of utopia in action. He believed in a foremost sense of duty over instinct and initiated and shepherded many utopian projects in the areas of education, alternative energy and artistic excellence.

Yehudiana, A new two part biography of Yehudi Menuhin by Philip Bailey documents these involvements in some detail.

For more information visit www.yehudiana.com

Foreword to the current edition

By Dr Donna Segal

As a Doctor of Audiology for 24 years, I understand the profound benefit of Sound Therapy. I am blessed to have come upon Patricia and Rafaele Joudry's mission through Sound Therapy. I have been using Sound Therapy for many years since I first became aware of their therapeutic treatment system.

Personally, I have experienced phenomenal mind, body and spiritual benefits from Sound Therapy. This ranges from alleviation of tinnitus in my left ear, fatigue, sinus and ear fullness, to concentration, improved sleep, reduction in severity of menopausal night sweats, TMJ and jaw stiffness, headache and neck tension and back pain. Listening to the system has allowed my body to hold my chiropractic adjustments longer as well as helped my muscles and co-ordination to flow more easily for yoga postures.

After becoming acquainted with Sound Therapy, I began studying the work of Dr. Alfred Tomatis. I became fascinated with his theories and the applications of this specially filtered music to healing the synergistic state of one's being. This was a wonderful complement to my audiological education and years of clinical practice in further understanding the hearing system. As I delved further into his work, I developed a deeper understanding of the ear and the perceptual connection, through the vital importance of Sound Therapy to even voice quality and production, reading and writing and overall emotional health.

I recommend and use Sound Therapy with my patients in my private practice. The benefits patients report range from reduction in sound sensitivity to improvement in sleep and energy as well as "just feeling better." As I continue to use this easy self-guided listening system all over the United States and Canada, I hear about its benefits to the overall consciousness of our planet. As people become more balanced and at harmony within themselves it expands outward to everyone they encounter.

I will continue to use Sound Therapy for the rest of my life. It has assisted me in helping release the lower frequency energy that our bodies tend to hold and then manifest in physical and emotional sensations — tinnitus being one of those. The benefits will vary for each individual person. Keep an open mind and attitude as you begin using the therapy, as you experience the release of patterns that may no longer serve your higher good, and as your system rebuilds more effective ear-brain connections. You will experience changes on many levels. Take your time moving through the program. As you move through reading this book and the workbook, you will notice the benefits within yourself.

I have used many different sound therapy systems on the market. I have found this Sound Therapy System easy to use. It has a broad range of benefits. Enjoy reading this book as Patricia Joudry takes you on a journey as she explains the Sound Therapy and its potential benefits and use. Whether you have specific challenges or just want to tune your system to optimal health, Sound Therapy is for you.

Donna Segal Au.D CCC-A
Doctor of Audiology
Sound Therapy Specialist in Private Practice
Perception Plus Inc.
Indianapolis, Indiana USA

Dr. Donna Segal holds a clinical doctorate in Audiology and has been studying the field of health and wellness for more than 25 years. She specialises in aural rehabilitation and works with individuals to allow them to retrain their brains to improve their overall perception. Dr. Segal's passion is helping others improve their health and well-being through nutrition and mind body welllness. She specialises in tinnitus and hyperacusis and teaches a tinnitus course at the doctorate level.

For further information visit www.perceptionplus.com

Introduction

By *Rafaele Joudry*

66 *He that hath ears to hear, let him hear.* 99

Matthew 11:15

Sometimes when they're happening we don't recognize those fateful moments that change the course of our lives. So it was the evening in Paris when I had a "chance" encounter with a Canadian Doctor who was there to study with Dr. Tomatis. I met this man, Gerard Binet, for a couple of minutes before going out with his flat-mate, and we idly chatted about what he was doing in Paris. Sound Therapy sounded rather intriguing. I'd never heard of being healed by sound! I almost didn't ask him if it would help my mother, but my friend took a little longer to get ready (the angels must have held him up,) so I thought "why not?" and I asked "would it help my mother?" I told him about my mother who had a peculiar (I thought then) condition of being unable to have a conversation if there was any background noise. (I have since learned that this condition, dubbed by audiologists "the cocktail party syndrome," is extremely common.)

Dr. Binet said with total confidence "Oh yes, it would cure that." I was rather surprised, but I got his number and wrote and told my mother. He was going back to open his Sound Therapy practice in Montreal where my mother lived, and it turned out she was one of his first clients.

The rest of the story is told in this book. The work of bringing Sound Therapy to the world in a compact, affordable and highly versatile package was laid out for my mother and me, or at least it was hanging on the branch of fate and we leaped and plucked it.

In my world travels I was guided to the next clue on our path. From

Paris I had moved out to Saskatchewan in Western Canada, and my mother had followed. It was there that she found the monks of St. Peters Abbey who helped her begin what became a life's work for both of us, though I was by then living in Australia.

When my mother sent me the first manuscript of this book, then entitled *Sound Therapy for the Walk Man* I read it with fascination and couldn't wait to try the program. I didn't have a problem like my mother's, but I nevertheless got benefit for my sleep and my general well-being. I slept more soundly the first night and I continued to use the program every night for seven years. Now I listen most days while working at the computer, on long trips or during a stressful period. Sound Therapy helps to restore my inner equilibrium, creativity and concentration, whilst refuelling my energy. I am a testament to the fact that even if you have no severe problems, the benefits offered by this therapy over a lifetime are still worth a gold mine.

We were initially amazed at the results achieved not only by my mother but by thousands of others. Listeners reported relief of tinnitus, better hearing, improved communication, and family relations, no more insomnia, dramatic increases in energy levels. People were being helped and the letters flooded in. Students claimed they could not have completed their degrees without Sound Therapy. Mothers told how their uncontrollable children had turned into little lambs and suddenly wanted to learn.

The therapy spread by word of mouth to forty-five countries in the first two years. When I saw the results others were having I realized this was too big a gift not to run with. So began my study of the ear, of tinnitus, chronic fatigue, ADHD, autism, speech problems and the many health and brain issues that Sound Therapy can help us address.

In 1993 I traveled across the United States and Canada and in New York met with Lynn Schroeder who, with Sheila Ostrander brought Superlearning to the West and wrote several best-selling books on advanced learning methods. Dr Lozanov, the father of accelerated learning, like Dr Tomatis, found a way of making classical music into a vitally healing tool for modern times. I have since met and formed collaborations with dozens of practitioners, doctors, audiologists, and others who enrich our understanding of how music impacts on the brain. This book, introducing our method, has continued to sell and to be loved by our readers. I have now brought the book up to date, adding several chapters of my own with references to current science, and contributions by those with relevant expertise.

I love working with this method because it empowers the individual by placing a powerfully healing tool in their own hands. The deeply gratifying gift of this work has been to receive people's feedback and to know that someone has overcome chronic pain, or tinnitus – that maddening condition of ringing in the ears – or the social isolation caused by a hearing disorder, or that their child is now learning to read as a result of the help Sound Therapy has given them. Some letters from our listeners follow.

Reports from Sound Therapy listeners

Jeff Johnson, Graduate Student, Dept. of Humanities, S.U.N.Y.,
Buffalo USA:

"Not only has Sound Therapy enhanced my learning capabilities, but it has greatly increased my confidence in speaking. Being a graduate student means that you must be able to speak with authority to groups of highly intelligent people. In the past I have been too shy and self-doubting to give such presentations with any confidence. They were the most anxiety-provoking situations of my life. My hands used to shake and I would be wet with perspiration before beginning to speak. Not anymore. I carry my Sound Therapy in my briefcase, and for a time before speaking I immerse myself in the recharging sounds of the music. I find then that I am perfectly at ease before large groups, and my presentations go without a hitch. Sound Therapy has helped me so much with my professional life that I've given it my own special name; I call it Confidence Therapy, because confidence was the area in which I was most lacking, and I now feel like a new man!"

Ed Rohner, President, United Fretters Ltd., Saskatoon Canada:

"The greatest benefit that Sound Therapy has had for me so far is in the area of hearing. I have a noticeable improvement in hearing and need less volume on my Walkman™ all the time. Also, I'm aware of having acquired the capacity for more highs. Most important of all for a musician, I am getting closer to pitch. I find I'm able to compensate the tuning which is required on any string instrument. With the increase in musical perception I am getting much more critical of sound. I firmly believe that a person who was tone deaf would be able to change that condition with Sound Therapy."

Judy and Gerrit Westerhof, Winnipeg Canada:

"Our son John is in Grade 6 and showing terrific improvement in reading since beginning on the Sound Therapy two months ago.

He says a lot of people don't even know he is dyslexic anymore. His teachers are amazed and thrilled, and even his friends have noticed the change in him. John came home last week and reported that two boys said, 'Boy, John, you're a lot smarter this year. Last year you were so dumb, but this year you're not.' We are so excited, because last year John was in a special program and this year he is in the regular program. He was on medication for his learning disability, but is now off the Ritalin. It makes him especially happy that he doesn't have to take the pills anymore, as they made him sick in his stomach. He loves the Baroque music, listening with his Auto-Reverse Walkman™ all night until the batteries run out. He hated to read before, and now when we have our evening devotions he asks to read and does it very well. It is like a miracle and he improves daily. His grandfather says it's like an alarm went off in his head and he woke up."

Lorna Graham, Hardings Point, Clifton Royal, NB, USA:

"I suffer from MS and have been listening to the Sound Therapy for about three months. I have had great luck in stabilizing my energy and can carry on normally. Nothing else I have done has helped me the way Sound Therapy has. The M stands for multiple or many, and so I need to do a lot of things, but the music really has helped bring it all together and make it worthwhile. It is a life-saver to me. It also keeps headaches at bay."

Dr. Kathleen Langston, Naramata, BC, Canada

"After 16 years of almost constant phantom pain due to amputation of my right leg from a car accident, I feel I have now found an answer. When I got my Sound Therapy I had some response almost at once, and it kept getting better. I didn't really believe it would help when I started; I had used so many things for phantom pain, even self-hypnosis, and had to take painkillers three or four times a day. Now I rarely take them, and only for some other complaint. The good results continue. It truly seems like a miracle."

Mrs. Gertrude Rempel Brown, Vancouver, Canada:

"It was pure accident that I heard Patricia Joudry being interviewed on radio. The word tinnitus caught my attention, and I began the Sound Therapy. My tinnitus, which my doctor said was incurable, was cured after several weeks of three hours a day listening. I had tinnitus for two years — and it was SHEER HEAVEN when it stopped — not to have incessant ringing in my ears. It also gives me a sense of well-being. I am lending the book to my doctor!"

Lorna Cooley, Victoria, BC, Canada:

"My husband suffered for many years with very bad headaches, which sometimes lasted for several days. Since receiving our Sound Therapy four months ago, we have each averaged more than four hours a day of listening. Since the first week or two my husband has not had any more of those headaches. It has also helped me, by lowering my blood pressure and giving me much more energy. My husband is 75 and I am 73. Your Sound Therapy sure is a gift for us older people, as well as the younger ones."

Marjorie Noyes, White Rock, BC, Canada:

"I have Parkinson's Disease. I lie down every day and put on my headphones and go into a very peaceful and restful sleep. I think Sound Therapy is beneficial for the stress that this malady brings on. Depression seems to be one of the worst side effects, and this is where Sound Therapy works wonders, making me feel reinforced to carry on my daily tasks."

Mrs. Marjorie Karpan, Keneston, Sask., Canada:

"I have noticed a remarkable change in my child's speech. The results were tremendous. The child is speaking in longer sentences, with more detail in speech. I am convinced that Sound Therapy really WORKS!"

Shirley Cowburn, Wigan, England:

"In addition to helping my tinnitus, the Sound Therapy made another wonderful difference in my life. My balance, which was very unsteady, following ear operations 30 years ago, has completely recovered, and this is marvellous for me and my family."

Margaret Owen, Balgowlah, NSW, Australia:

"Three days after beginning Sound Therapy I travelled by coach to Brisbane, normally an exhausting procedure, playing the music throughout the journey – slept soundly and arrived full of energy into heat-wave conditions – and spent the afternoon sight-seeing at a rapid pace.

The second benefit was being able to cut my sleeping time down to seven hours per night for the first time in my life, thus enabling me to get more done. The extra energy has been such a bonus that I don't care about the acuity of my hearing though I'm sure it's much improved.

I don't go anywhere without my Walkman, Sound Therapy and battery charger. Even walking round the city is not the exhausting experience it used to be."

Gladys Irwin, West Pennant Hills NSW, Australia:

"After a hearing test three years ago, I was fitted with hearing aids, which proved helpful. After several months the tinnitus in the right ear was so strong that the aid was useless.

When I learned about Sound Therapy I purchased the book which I found fascinating, so I tried the program. For eight months I have persevered with the treatment. In the last three months I realised my hearing had improved so that I can now do without the aids.

This was confirmed recently when I was examined by an ear, nose and throat specialist, who said that I had the hearing of a woman forty – I am eighty-seven!

Now I can hear the Bell Birds unaided."

Updates

A note on language and technology

In this revised edition, in certain cases, words referring to superceded formats such as tape and cassette have been changed to avoid confusion.

Be sure to follow the recommendations from Sound Therapy International for current technology and playback formats. Never try to copy or download Sound Therapy albums as this will reduce or destroy the therapeutic effect.

Always listen to Sound Therapy in its original format as supplied by Sound Therapy International.

For more information visit: www.SoundTherapyInternational.com

Changing technology and Sound Therapy

When Sound Therapy was first invented by Dr. Alfred Tomatis in the 1950's it was delivered to the listener through headphones directly from reel to reel tapes in the clinic. In 1984, when Patricia Joudry developed the portable system, this was possible due to the recent invention of the Sony Walkman and metallic cassettes which gave us the first high quality portable audio.

Since then most audio playback has converted to digital methods, some of which use compressed, low quality formats not suitable for Sound Therapy.

Sound Therapy International ensures that the program is made available on the best, most current high quality portable format. Check with your Sound Therapy consultant or company website for the current program, format and equipment.

IMPORTANT: Never attempt to make copies of Sound Therapy albums as this will down grade the integrity and quality of the specially processed high frequency sound.

Updated references for this edition

The book has been completely revised for this 12th edition to bring the information up to date. As part of this process I have added references to the parts written by my mother. Some of these references may have been published after the original book was written, as I have endeavoured, without changing her original message and themes, to elucidate cases where more recent research may have confirmed or added to the original theories presented here.

Spelling

As this book is intended for supply internationally in America, Australia and Europe, for a number of words I have used American spellings. My apologies to English and Australian readers.

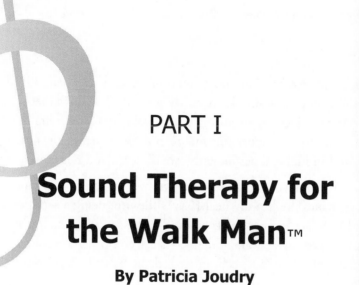

PART I

Sound Therapy for the Walk Man™

By Patricia Joudry

Chapter One

The Sound Effect

 There are sounds which are as good as two cups of coffee
Dr. Alfred Tomatis

It's called Audio-Psycho-Phonology but don't let that scare you. Like all great discoveries it is simple. According to Dr. Tomatis's theory, The brain is recharged by means of sound, releasing latent vitality, obliterating tiredness, heightening mental powers, lessening the need for sleep, and inducing a permanent state of peace and relaxation.

It is a therapy, but you needn't be ill. Known generally as Sound Therapy, it makes the healthy healthier, while producing a series of benefits almost as varied as the brain itself. The sound is the music of Mozart, Haydn, Bach and other classical composers, recorded by a special high frequency technique, and the method is the Sony Walkman™.[1]

You listen while walking, or reading, driving, shopping, riding the subway or plane, talking, even sleeping. If you're a student you listen and benefit while studying, if you're a monk, while praying, if an artist, while writing or painting.

Until recently Sound Therapy has been used only for the treatment of disorders. The principles were evolved by Dr. A. A. Tomatis of Paris, a former ear, nose and throat specialist whose investigations into the effect of sound upon the human mind have brought him high honour and recognition. The therapy has been used in Europe for more than three decades, achieving positive results with hearing disorders, emotional disturbance, hypertension, insomnia,

---

1   At the time of first writing, the cassette Walkman was the method used for playback, but portable music technology has changed since then. Contact Sound Therapy International for the latest updates.

speech defects, epilepsy, hyperactivity, dyslexia, and even autism.[2] Essentially, the treatment consists of listening, through headphones, to high frequency music recorded through a device of Tomatis's invention known as the Electronic Ear. The music is called 'filtered', because the low frequencies have been filtered out, leaving only the highs, or recharging sounds.

For decades, the cost in time and money had limited the benefit to those in urgent need, the patient being required to sit for several hours a day connected by headphones to the highly sophisticated equipment in the therapist's listening room. There, the filtered music was relayed via reel-to-reel tapes played through the Electronic Ear. Now a way has been found to put the sound program onto portable music players.

The big advantage of the portable system is the freedom of movement it affords the listener, and thus the great saving in time. The advent of portable audio, which began with the Sony Walkman™, has made Sound Therapy available to the majority, which means the healthy, more or less. Every one of us is subject to stresses. Now, instead of reaching for the valium or the scotch – or somebody's throat – we can reach for the headphones and find calm as well as resurgent energy. Paradoxically, this restorative sound vitalizes while it relaxes. Working directly upon the cortex of the brain, it mobilizes the complementary forces of the human system and, certainly in my own experience, provides a natural high and a natural sedative, each coming into play at the dictate of the will.

Each person is a centre of energy, continually influenced by other energies, light and colour and sound. Of these, the most powerful is sound.[3] Poets and mystics speak of the music of the spheres, and we know that the universe is created upon mathematical principles and that mathematics and music have the same root. Some theologians believe that the statement, 'In the beginning was the Word' points to sound as the first creative principle. For once they are not divided

2   Tomatis, A.A., The Conscious Ear, Station Hill Press, New York, 1991.
3   Berendt, Joachim. E., *The Third Ear*. New York: Henry Holt & Company Inc. New York, 1992.

from the scientists who claim it all began with a big bang. Maybe it will end with one too, as a demonstration of the difference between sound and noise.

Noise can damage our hearing

Noise is unwanted sound and is the curse of our day. The populations of entire countries are in danger of suffering hearing losses due to the increasing mechanization of society. The ear, the most sensitive organ in human or animal, is the first to respond to its surroundings. Anyone who has watched a mouse be subjected for a few seconds to the sound of a siren and subsequently suffer a convulsive audiogenic attack that can be fatal, understands that noise is not merely an unpleasant sensation or a danger for the structure of the ear; it is the most important factor in disequilibrium, the great poison that intoxicates the nerve centres at the base of the brain.

Prolonged exposure to noise of 85 decibels or higher produces permanent hearing loss, and traffic noises at that db level are common for the city dweller.[4] Subways and airports have noise levels of 93 and 130 db respectively. One motorcycle generates the same sound hazard as 100 automobiles.

We are passive victims of this noise. There is no protection except to stay in bed with a pillow over our head. The best that the medical profession can do for us is hand out advice like: "Noise-induced hearing loss can be limited by the wearing of ear plugs, by periodic audiometric examination to detect early changes in hearing acuity" (then what?) "and by the environmental control of noise." Have you tried controlling noise in your environment lately? Throwing a shoe out the window at a motorcycle is about the extent of our power.

---

4   "Types of Hearing Loss." *Dangerous Decibels: a public health partnership for the prevention of noise induced hearing loss.* Cited on 13th Sept 2009 http://www.dangerousdecibels.org/hearingloss.cfm

DECIBEL COMPARISON CHART

Loud sound has a cumulative effect and can permanently damage hearing. Noise levels are measured in decibels (dB). The higher the decibel level, the louder the noise. Sounds louder than 80 decibels are considered potentially hazardous. This chart indicates average decibel levels for everyday sounds around you.

Faint

30 dB = whisper, quiet library

Moderate

40 dB = quiet room

50 dB = moderate rainfall

60 dB = dishwasher

60-70 dB = normal conversation

Very Loud

70 dB = busy traffic, vacuum cleaner

80 dB = alarm clock, busy street

80 dB = telephone dial tone

82-92 dB = violin

Extremely Loud

Level at which sustained exposure may result in hearing loss

90 dB = lawnmower, shop tools, truck traffic

90-106 = French horn

95 dB = subway train

100 dB = snowmobile, chain saw, pneumatic drill

106 dB = timpani and bass drum rolls

107 dB = power mower

110 dB = rock music, model airplane

Painful

Even short-term exposure can cause permanent damage

120 dB = jet plane take-off, amplified rock music at 4-6 ft., car stereo, band practice

120-137 dB = symphonic music peak

130 dB = jackhammer

140 dB = firearms, air raid siren, jet engine

150 dB = rock music peak

Sound Therapy: our choice

Now at last it is possible to select the influence to which we want to expose our ear and brain. The noise of the world can't be drowned out, but it can be defused by a gentle sound that we may carry with us anywhere. The high frequency music may serve to protect our hearing over the long term by providing needed stimulation to brain pathways in the auditory cortex. Deterioration usually begins with the sensory hair cells in the basal portion of the cochlea which reduces sensitivity to the higher frequencies first; and that is the area which is rehabilitated by the listening therapy.

The self-therapy requires nothing more than that we listen, through earphones for a period each day to the pleasant, specially processed classical music. We needn't even listen consciously, but can set the Walkman™ at low volume and go on with whatever we're doing. The effect is of a recharge to the brain, resulting in a release of energy throughout the body.

The role of the human ear

Tomatis's great contribution to science was to define the role that the ear plays in relation to the human body. He tells us that the ear is made not only for hearing, but is intended to benefit the organism by the stimulation of sound. It can be shown by electroencephalography that the brain uses energy. This electricity is engendered by the central grey nuclei, which are like batteries constantly recharging. The energy which is discharged can be captured. These outbursts of activity do not arise from metabolic processes but from the stimulation of this area by the external input. The battery is recharged via the ear. There are 24,600 sensory cells on the level of the basilar membrane's organ of corti, and these cells are accumulated particularly in the zone of the high frequencies. If one augments the capacity of recharging, via auditory input at high frequencies, the richest area of the basilar membrane is stimulated, as these special nuclei of the cortex are the ones which are more energy-laden.

It is not simply a matter of exposing the ear to high frequencies. We are not accustomed to tuning in to these frequencies and won't be capable of filtered-music recharge until the doors leading to the inner ear are opened. A re-education of the middle ear is required, and for this purpose the music is recorded through Tomatis's Electronic Ear.

Tomatis's Electronic Ear

This complex machine constitutes the essence of the treatment. The device is set to a specific algorithm, which selectively filters bass and treble sounds. The output is a series of tones in particular frequency ranges, which act dynamically to retrain the hearing pathways between the ear and brain. The patterns of alternating frequencies which are related to and embedded in the complex structure of the classical music cause the middle ear muscles to alternately tense and relax in a rocking motion.[5] The pattern of tension and relaxation acts as a gymnastic and conditions the musculature so that later it will have the ability to regulate the action itself.[6] The spikes and changes in the sound pattern provide a unique stimulation to the brain. Over time more accurate pathways are built so that faithful perception of sound will become habitual. The ear will have discovered its full listening function and its power to vitalize the brain. This process has undergone changes and modifications over the years, as we added to and improved on Tomatis's original knowledge base.

As sound is transformed into nervous influx the charge of energy to the cortex is distributed throughout the nervous system, imparting greater dynamism to the person and flowing into all the areas of need. Like the healing energy of the flesh, mental energy is entirely beneficent, enhancing the creativity of the artist, soothing the insomniac to sleep while rousing the lethargic, harmonizing the

---

5   Tomatis, A.A., *The Conscious Ear*, Station Hill Press, New York, 1991.
6   Weeks, Bradford S., "The Therapeutic Effect of High Frequency Audition and its Role in Sacred Music"; *About the Tomatis Method*, eds. Gilmor, Timothy M., Ph.D., Madaule, Paul, L.Ps., Thompson, Billie, Ph.D. The Listening Centre Press, Toronto, 1989. Article can be cited on http://weeksmd.com/?p=714 Also see Appendix.

disturbed pathways in the brain which have caused speech and learning defects, uplifting the depressive, and in some instances opening the autistic child to human connection.[7]

About Sound Therapy

It takes time for Sound Therapy to recharge the brain

Involving as it does a rehabilitation of the ear, Sound Therapy is a process requiring a certain length of time. The effect of the music will not be immediate. On an average, 100 to 200 hours of listening are necessary before there is a noticeable change in the energy level and sense of well-being. But once the middle ear has been tuned to high frequency response the brain will respond swiftly to the recharge. If you happen to have gone out without your Walkman™ and arrive home tired, ten minutes' relaxation with the music will be like hours of sleep. Eventually, with regular recharging, you will forget what tiredness was like.

Perhaps the greatest bounty of the Tomatis Effect is its gift of time. Once the opening of the auditory system has occurred, some listeners report that sleep can safely be reduced by one, two or three hours a night, with the waking time becoming more vital and useful. Energy never flags, yet peace and relaxation permeate the hours. This is our own natural energy which has been blocked and is now restored. [8]

Academic recognition for Tomatis's methods

It sounds like magic and it is, magic being simply natural law not previously understood. Tomatis's work is thoroughly scientific; his discoveries have been tested and confirmed by the Sorbonne University in Paris, and given the name The Tomatis Effect. As a result he has been made a member of the French Academy of Medicine and the Academy of Science.

Distinctions awarded to Tomatis as recognition of his early work were

---

7   Tomatis, A.A., *The Conscious Ear*, Station Hill Press, New York, 1991.
8   Tomatis, A.A., Ibid.

as follows: Chavalier of public health 1951; International Scientific Research Gold Medal at the Brussels World Fair (1959) awarded for the Tomatis Effect Electronic Ear; International Scientific Research Bronze Medal at the Brussels World Fair (1959) for the Tomatis Automatic Audiometer; Grande Medaille de Vermail of the City of Paris (1962); Clemence Isaure Prize. March 1967; Arts, Science and Literature Gold medal, April 1968.

Counteracting hearing distortions

Everyone is restricted to some extent by blockages arising from distortions of hearing. During their early years, in order not to hear certain unpleasant sounds, Tomatis says that children may deafen themselves in the area of high frequencies, cut off their auditory diaphragm and withdraw from communication by involuntarily choosing longer brain circuits. They then lose much of their potential, particularly the ability to listen to language; in extreme cases they may develop dyslexia or other disorders which baffle diagnosis. Tomatis, who discovered for us the strict relationship that exists between our mental attitude and our listening, has successfully treated more than 12,000 subjects for dyslexia by transforming the receptivity of the ear. He found that if there is a failure of hearing at a certain low point of frequency, all the areas above that frequency will be blocked. But when the ear is re-educated and the barrier is lifted, below for instance 1,000 Hz, all the other areas wake up very quickly and the subject is able to benefit from the store of vitality which has been dormant.[9]

We have to distinguish between charging sounds, those rich in high harmonics, and the low, or discharging sounds. In the region of 3,000 to 20,000 Hz, sound mainly serves the function of producing cortical arousal, whereas low frequencies tend to exhaust the system; they can actually be dangerous, as they demand of the body a greater discharge of energy than the cortex receives in stimulation. The sound of the tom-tom, for example, is intended specifically to make

---

9   Tomatis, A.A., Ibid.

the body move and to send the listeners into a secondary state, a sort of hypnosis, which puts them at the mercy of more powerful minds, such as the witch doctor's. High frequency sounds, on the other hand, lead the subject to consciousness and self-actualization.

The implication at the psycho-dynamic level is that depressive persons tend to direct their hearing more intensely toward low frequencies; and, as the voice is directly related to the ear, often speak in a low monotone. The ear has lost its ability, suggests Tomatis, to be used as an antenna for the life force.

The recharging effect of high frequency sounds

In contrast to a depressed person, the person whose ear has been trained to high frequencies begins tuning into these recharging sounds in the surrounding air, drawing upon an unending source of energy and upliftment. Among all professions, the people with the greatest longevity are orchestral conductors, who spend the greater part of their waking hours in direct exposure to classical music, the type of music that contains the greatest percentage of frequencies.

Tomatis says: "What the youth of today is looking for is the stimulation of their brain. The trouble is that they are taken up not with charging sounds but with discharging sounds. In the music they play there are no high harmonics. The more they play, the more tired they feel, and the more they are obliged to increase the intensity. That music discharges you; it compels the organism into mechanical movement. Such involvement taxes the musculature without recharging the organism."

It is impossible to be in good health when brain systems are not in proper working order, yet the very idea of the brain makes people nervous. "So little is known about the brain," we are told, and the implications are ominous. All this mystery makes the brain seem as scary as a haunted house; we're afraid to even look in the window, let alone stir things up.

"Recharge the brain?" said one man in alarm. "What happens when the brain can't be recharged any more?"

Well, the time comes for every brain when it can't be recharged any more. It's called death. Until then our brains are continually being charged or discharged by the sounds around us, and we'd be wise to determine what those sounds are going to be, while we still have the brain to do it with. Unless it is kept toned up, the brain merely deteriorates with the advance of years, and there lies the root problem of old age. The real heartbreak for the aged is feeling themselves a burden to others. But you can bet that all branches of the family would be fighting over who was going to have Grandma or Grandpa if these were sparkling companions, full of fresh ideas and wit and the health that is controlled by the master computer of the body. This stage of life awaits us all. Instead of (or along with) the savings in the bank to allow independence when we become a drag, it would be worth our while to accumulate the more fundamental currency of life energy which flows in to us through the brain.

We needn't fear using that energy up like our oil resources. Nowhere is it written: "This much and no more you may have." This is the energy of the cosmos, continually passing through us – or trying to. More often it can't break in and has to surge round us like water round an obstacle in the river. It is all available, if we'll just let it in. Yoga exercises teach us how to bring it into our muscles. Toning the cortex is no different from toning the muscles.

Such toning, with its effect upon the frontal lobes which regulate attention and concentration, makes the therapy particularly valuable for students. Words and ideas are more readily absorbed and retained, and also the power of creativity is heightened. The increase in cortical energy permits the person's thoughts to be expressed more easily, in various creative forms. Through the action upon the basilar membrane, rich in sensory fibres, general perception is improved and the body image harmonized.

Sound Therapy for healing past traumas

It should be emphasized that the electronic technique is in no way designed to condition the subject artificially. It is not intended

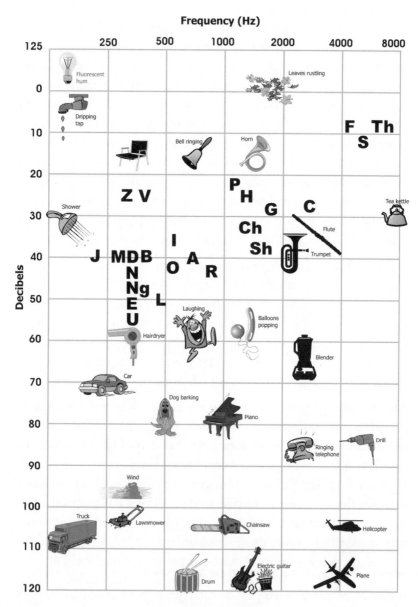

Diagram of Sounds

to conform the ears and the brain, but merely to assist in the full opening of auditory perceptions, so that persons who are traumatized, frustrated or restricted by incidents in their history, may regain the positive freedom of their nature. The maladjustments which have caused a partial closing of the ear tend toward a partial closing of the personality to other people and to the world in general. The therapy has broad psychological applications and fortifies the principles of psychoanalysis, while streamlining the process. Both have the same goal, to obtain the greatest possible maturing of the person. While it takes a great deal of time to be freed of complexes through psychoanalysis, Sound Therapy arrives at the same result by a more direct route, bringing about the maturation of the individual by working directly on the brain structures.

Dr. Sarkissof, a psychoanalyst, speaking at the International Congress of the SECRAP in 1972, describes certain patients whom he had agreed to analyze, rather reluctantly, not holding a great deal of hope for their cure. He states:

"The results of these analyses confirmed my doubts as to the possibility of completely curing these patients. The more time passed the more I doubted that I could succeed in obtaining anything more than an improvement of their condition – I decided to let them undergo treatment with the Tomatis apparatus. Not only did they accept willingly, but they accepted with gratitude and high hopes, and I realized, although they had not spoken of it, that all of them were fully aware that treatment by psychoanalysis alone could not completely cure them. The material they offered at the sessions then changed radically. In each of them the Tomatis apparatus brought to light fantasies of a return to the mother's breast and to birth, and the analysis of these fantasies was accompanied by a clearly visible transformation of their entire personality. All these patients shared a core of unconscious autism: their emotional contacts were without warmth and life, their analyses went round in circles without uncovering any particular cause of resistance, which meant a basic difficulty in communication. Sound Therapy rapidly reduced this core of autism. In the space of a few months, the autism gave way to a joyful, outgoing self-awareness, and their co-operation in the analysis became fruitful. My personal reservations regarding these patients gave way to great optimism as to their ability to get well completely. One of the patients expressed his astonishment at noting that he had suddenly become capable of making great progress, readily and without anxiety, while he remembered that before the treatment, the efforts demanded of him in psychoanalysis seemed immense and completely out of proportion to the slight progress he made. He considered the Tomatis treatment a very valuable short cut, which made him feel that he was making a game of his difficulties."

Dr. Sarkissof explains that our destiny is recorded somewhere inside us as if on a magnetic tape which preserves the memory of what we experience. This store, in turn, plays a determining role in our process of becoming. None of our actions is indifferent but each affects the future, as we constantly recreate ourselves. A magnetic tape is not erased automatically. A special device is required. Thus it is very difficult to erase from our mind the tapes of our past which are recorded in our subconscious. "We have two methods for bringing this about," continues Dr. Sarkissof. "One consists of bringing it onto the conscious level; that is into the present. This is the method of psychoanalysis. It is often very lengthy and demands much courage and perseverance. The Tomatis apparatus brings us another method. It succeeds in erasing the 'tape' without bringing it into the conscious mind. It can eliminate for the patient the suffering of reliving his neurosis. During the treatment he continues to unwind the tape of his life without difficulty. The traumatic experiences of his past are erased from his subconscious directly, for the Tomatis treatment has the advantage of reaching the deepest layers of the subconscious, liberating him from fixations and eliminating the obstacles to normal functioning. The personality is then free to develop unhindered and recover the subconscious energy which was blocked."

The same applies for the mildly neurotic and for those who are reasonably healthy, like the rest of us. We do the listening for simple brain recharge, yet as our control centres are harmonized, things sort themselves out at deep levels without us ever having to know what they are – or admit they were there. The complex is made simple – a rare occurrence in our desperate and complicated time.

Audio-Psycho-Phonology is a cybernetic system of appalling complexity, and the literature is enough to stagger the mind. Yet when it comes to the practice the complexities don't matter. It's like electricity: you don't have to understand the principle behind it in order to light your room; all you have to know is how to put in a light bulb and flick a switch. To reap the benefits of Sound Therapy you only have to slip on your headphones. And the expenditure in time is absolutely nothing. With the convenience and portability of the Walkman™ you can do the complete listening program while continuing all your usual activities – with a few exceptions like tennis and sex.

Sound Therapy: Comparing the original and the portable methods

The above discussion doesn't mean that listening to Sound Therapy will cure everything, or that it will do the same thing as the original Tomatis therapy. Serious problems will require the skills of a trained therapist. The Tomatis equipment conveys a higher frequency than a portable player, and the Tomatis trained therapists have other techniques to go with it. The self-conducted portable system has two main advantages. It makes this great discovery available in some measure to the many instead of the few. And the effects, while they take longer to achieve, can be maintained, in that the person can keep up the listening for months, years, or for life, as most satisfied subjects are resolved to do.

Another consideration is the cost. The price of the portable program is a fraction of what people pay for most therapies. And the will power required is minimal compared to analysis or even meditation.

In fact Sound Therapy is the perfect therapy for those who find it hard to get motivated.

Accepting the filtered music

Still, there must be a sputter of life in the resolve to undertake the daily listening and to accept that the sound is not exactly the same thing as having the best seat at a concert. Some people don't like the high pitched sound of filtered music, though others find it very pleasant. It may be that tolerance is directly related to the desire for self-betterment. Certainly, those who unconsciously desire to hang on to their deafness or sleeplessness or perpetual tiredness are going to object to the sound. In contrast are those self-improvers who become positively addicted to it and lose all interest in 'normal' music. Said one, "I start listening to my regular music and soon realize it's not doing anything for me. It's like drinking a highball when you forgot to put in the liquor."

Not that the Tomatis effect bears any relation to the liquor effect. The difference between the alcohol high and this one is that the Sound Therapy lift is healthy and it stays with you. It is a boost onto a higher level in the domain of our vast, unrealized potential. Drink fuzzes the mind, while these filtered sounds clarify it to a high sheen. One person has described the sensation as "like having a new head." Another feels as though her mind had been put through a shower.

Positive side effects of Sound Therapy

As the headphones are lifted off after a half hour or so, there is a glowing feeling between the ears, a sense of radiant energy, not the revved-up energy of the chemical high, but a calm and peaceful aliveness, as in those moments when we are very happy, having just had good news, or simply being tuned to the joy of life.

Sound therapists have known that their treatment of various disorders brings wonderful "side effects" in the form of energy and well-being. For the healthy person these constitute a major effect.

But healthy people are not in the habit of seeking treatment to maintain their good condition and raise it to sparkling – though they do it regularly for their cars.

Who would think of going to a sound therapist and saying: "I don't need the treatment, but I'd like the side effects please"? For that matter, who, when I lived in Canada in the late 1970s would have thought of going to a sound therapist? Sound therapists could be counted on the fingers of one hand then and they were promoted as little as Canadian writers.

But this Canadian writer stumbled over one like a treasure in the dark, and so is obeying the universal rule of supply, which dictates:

Pass it on.

Chapter Two

Plugged into the Cosmos

> ❝ *If you put an oscilloscope on the sounds of Gregorian Chant,* ❞
> *you see that they all come within the bandwidth for*
> *charging the ear.*
>
> Dr. Alfred Tomatis

Looking back, it doesn't seem strange that I should have been one of the first people in the country to find my way to a sound therapist's door, as most of my life has been lived off the beaten track. For example, you can read about my experiment in allowing my children to educate themselves at home (as distinct from 'educating' them at home) if you care to see my book, *And the Children Played*, reprinted by Tundra Books, Montreal, Spring, '84.

One of these children, Rafaele (formerly Melanie), having graduated from college (her first experience of school) was continuing her self-education and spending the year 1977 in Paris to perfect her French. There, by chance as they call it, she met a French-Canadian doctor who was studying Sound Therapy with Dr. Tomatis. Rafaele spoke to him about her mother's hearing problem, a matter of great inconvenience to the family, though they were always very nice about it.

My anti-social hearing problem

My problem was this: I couldn't carry on a conversation if there were other people talking in the room. If I had to talk against the voice background, or listen to someone speaking to me, the cross vibrations of sound simply broke up my focus. At home I was constantly calling for silence and then trying to get a single conversation going while everybody else held their tongues. It was socially debilitating, to say the least, and it was getting worse. At a publisher's party for one of my books I had to sneak out after a few minutes and go home. Luckily there was lots to drink and I never did hear that anybody noticed.

I had mentioned this malady to a number of people who told me they had it too. So of course the Canadian doctor recognized it at once from the description. He told my daughter that it could be cured with Sound Therapy. She asked him what Sound Therapy was, and considering the explanation that found its way back to me, it's a good thing I go on faith.

Accordingly, when he returned to Montreal to set up practice the following spring, I was right there. We had a nice talk, (no-one else was speaking in the room) and a few days later my treatment commenced.

The listening test

All was mystery from the word go, and the word was not "Go," it was "Beep." Connected by headphones to an unearthly looking machine, on which the therapist produced high-pitched sounds by twirling a handle, I had to state when I heard what, and where. During all this he was drawing a graph with coloured pencils. I felt strangely elated by these high tones and attributed it to the total yogic concentration necessary to decide whether they came from right, left or centre. I was also asked whether a sequence of sounds was getting higher or lower. They were all sky high and sometimes I just didn't know. I gave answers, then took them back. It was like sitting for an examination that I didn't want to fail.

The headphones were changed for another pair that didn't go on my ears at all. They fitted over the mastoid bone and the bone at my temple. I was amazed to find that I could hear through my bones as well as through my ears. It was the first I knew of the fact that we hear with our whole body. This was downtown Montreal and the traffic sounds outside were like an artillery attack. They had devastated me previously and were now made harmless by these eloquent little electronic bleeps. I could hardly believe my ears – or my ears could scarcely believe the soothing yet stimulating sound that promised an end to abuse.

When the listening test was completed, the therapist was able to view the precise nature of my trouble. He saw another one that I hadn't thought to mention for how could it relate to sound? It was my complete helplessness at all things technical. Like a clairvoyant he read this from the graph. It was absolutely true. I could barely change a light bulb, couldn't possibly replace a fuse, and always had to get some small child to put in my typewriter ribbon. On the day the stereo system was delivered and the kids were showing me how to use it, I am quoted as saying: "Oh, I have to press Stop? I'll never be able to work that." The family was still laughing. (But the last laugh would be mine.)

Next, the therapy was explained to me – in simple words, with respect to my deficiencies in the technical field. As it is quite impossible to really put across the principles of Sound Therapy in simple words, I again had to take it on faith. It seemed that a specific listening program would be designed for me.

Listening subconsciously

My listening program would consist largely of the music of Mozart, and I would sit and listen to it for three hours every week-day during the next six weeks.

"That's all?" I asked. "There's nothing more to it?"

"Yes. Bring some sewing or embroidery to work on. It's better to absorb the sound subconsciously, with the attention fixed on something else."

It turned out that women patients did needlework and men did jigsaw puzzles. I was gladder than ever to be a female.

Game for anything, I settled into the routine, driving the sixty miles from my farm at St. Agnes de Dundee and sitting for three hours daily, comfortably settled in an armchair in a little room, with my headphones, my sewing and my thermos of tea. The music was recognizably Mozart, though Mozart would have had a fit. The violin concertos, symphonies and chamber pieces all started out normally, except for occasional soft hissing sounds. Then, imperceptibly, the lower sounds began giving way to the strings. After a time even the strings were clinging to the rafters. It was strange, eerie, and perversely pleasing. Yet I wondered. It just didn't seem possible that sitting here listening to squeaky music for three hours was going to relieve me of anything but thirty-six dollars. (By now the fee is considerably higher, all low prices having been filtered out everywhere!)

The equipment from which all this originated was stacked in the next room and operated by an assistant. It looked pretty spooky with its blinking lights and turning reels, and I always hurried past it, while noting that wires snaked under several doors to other patients in their comfy little dens. It was good to know that others were willing to take a chance, though when I stopped to think of it, I never saw them. I pondered about what their personalized listening programs might be like while I imbibed the one specifically designed to sort out the crossed wires in my head – or whatever it was that so inhibited the social life I didn't much want. I was really doing this from a fear that my hearing quirk might lead to deafness. I had seen my mother gradually lose her hearing and become isolated from human company and, almost worse, from music. Nietzche put his finger on it when he said: "Without music life would be a mistake."

I stuck this out week after week, trying lamely to explain at home the purpose of the daily trek. They surmised that Sound Therapy was some kind of faith healing. If that's what it was it wouldn't work, because I was starting to lose faith. Also, there was no sign of healing. I observed my reactions with mounting anxiety, like a hypochondriac taking her own pulse every few minutes. I was neither better nor worse. I began to resent the time that was going into this. And the car was eating up a lot of gas.

The fourth week offered a little variety in the form of a vocalizing technique. A microphone was set up on the table in my little room and a new tape relayed through the headphones. A female voice gave instructions, then spoke sibilant words at high frequency, leaving a gap between each. In the gap I was to repeat the word into the microphone. As I did this, my own voice, also filtered to very high pitch, came back into my ears. Due to past experience as a radio actress I felt quite at home with the mike, though I never expected to be presented with a script like this.

Next, a monk with a beautiful voice came on singing phrases of Gregorian chant, with cathedral echo backup. He too waited for my repetition, and I was glad he couldn't hear it, for I never could carry a tune.

It was all terribly wearing. A deep exhaustion settled over me. My therapist had warned that I might get a little tired: it would mean that the therapy was working, the effect beginning to be felt in the muscle of the middle ear, the brain patterns rearranging themselves. He explained it again. I couldn't follow any of it. I hadn't the strength. The exhaustion that had seeped into me could only be compared with the depleted feeling that follows childbirth – or finishing a novel. Arriving home at night after the sixty-mile drive, I could hardly drag myself out of the car. I detested driving anyway; cars were technical and I hated them.

A calm sense of energy

How did it begin? I first noticed it at the wheel, while stopped in the rush-hour traffic. It was a kind of gentle vibration in my head, a sense of something about to take off. I began singing, using the humming technique I had learned in my sessions. I sang my way out of Montreal and hummed as I spun along the highway. When I got home I noted with surprise that I was not tired. Far from it.

I stayed up late doing things around the house, and rose early the next morning, deeply rested and refreshed. The effect was subtle – not a high-powered charge but a sure, calm sense of energy. It was energy formerly untapped, now available, ready to be drawn upon as needed. The feeling of well-being increased day by day, peaking at moments – usually in the evening when I would ordinarily be flaked out – and sending a dynamism sparking along my veins as though I were electrically connected. I told my therapist: "I feel as though I've been plugged into the cosmos."

He only smiled. He knew about this. For one thing he had taken the therapy himself in France as part of his training. His serenity was one of the characteristic results. Yet I saw him excited too – on the day when he opened the door of another listening room and pointed to a child wearing headphones and stretched out on a sofa.

"That child," he told me softly, "was so hyper that his parents were going to have to institutionalize him. Now he lies still for three hours every day listening to Mozart." Later the boy's mother also came for treatment, and the family found harmony.

Within a week I was going around in a perpetual state of exultation. Before my therapy began I'd been working on a novel. It had struck a roadblock and stopped. Suddenly the words began flowing again. I sat scribbling all through my sessions and was still working at home at midnight, though ordinarily I wasn't able to write beyond noon. (That book was *The Selena Tree*, published by McClelland and Stewart, now in a New Canadian Library paperback edition. You might note the dedication.)

I seemed to feel no need for sleep. When I went to bed it was not because I was tired, but because the next day had rolled around and I thought I ought to. For years I had had difficulty sleeping and had made a huge point of going to bed at nine, to read for an hour and toss around for another two, so as to be asleep by midnight and get the eight hours I needed for a good morning's work. This meant I had no evenings and neither did the others in the house, who had to tiptoe around and keep their talk to a whisper. Now I was seeing them off to bed while I charged around the house, typing, cooking, cleaning, catching up on correspondence and all those things which drag at the mind. When I lay down to sleep – miraculously, I slept.

My problem cured

On an afternoon in my sixth and final week, as I sat listening in my little room, the therapist came strolling in. I tensed up, in mortal fear that he was going to say something. Not only did I have to keep silent when there were voices in the background, but also when music was playing.

He began to speak. I went into my act, waving my hands frantically and objecting: "I've got the music on! I can't talk when there's music on, I never could!"

He smiled and said calmly: "You can now."

I stopped short and listened to him. I ventured to answer. We chatted about many things and the music played on, and he was right: I had been cured.

I went out into the stores and talked to salespeople, with the babble of voices all around me. No problem. I couldn't believe it. Neither could my family when I got home that night. I walked into the house and all talk stopped, as usual.

"Go right on," I said airily. "Doesn't bother me a bit."

Now I became intensely curious as to what had happened. I had asked several times: "What does the sound do exactly?" and could never understand the answer. It couldn't be told in a few sentences. (One would have to write a book!) It had to do with recharging the cortex of the brain and was accompanied by some sort of theory about a return to the womb and a rebirth through sound. This clarified the picture for me as much as seeing it through water.

"It works," the therapist said. "That's what counts."

It was true. From that day to this I have never been troubled by cross-currents of voices – though my daughters were disappointed about the paper bags. You see, along with everything else, my hearing has always been very acute, and there was something about the resonating crackle of paper bags being folded that struck my eardrums like spears. On shopping day, therefore, as we unpacked the groceries, I was always warning: "Don't fold the bags till I'm out." I finally left the kitchen awash in open, empty paper bags!

So the girls had hoped my therapy would take care of this too. But the effect of the sound is to open the hearing – so it was worse with the bags. Nothing's perfect.

As the day approached when my listening sessions were to end, I began to feel bereft. What if it all wore off? I asked my therapist – I begged him: "Isn't there some way I could listen to this kind of music at home?"

He assured me there wasn't. "You would have to buy all this." He waved at the equipment. "It cost twenty thousand dollars."

If I'd had the twenty thousand, I'd have spent it on that in a minute.

"Even then," he went on, "you wouldn't know how to use it."

That was certainly true. And given the state of technological development at that time, he was right that there was no way. He wasn't lying to me. He just didn't know he was talking to someone at whom the eye of fate had just winked.

After the final session he gave me the listening test again, and showed me on the graph the changes that had taken place. I didn't have to see the graph. A graph is only two-dimensional lines. I knew in all the complex dimensions of myself the transformation that had occurred. I hugged him wordlessly and left. I felt strangely alone, unconnected from the equipment.

As the weeks passed, I slowly became unconnected from the cosmos too. The radiant energy flickered and faded. At the end of the day I was tired like anybody else. Sleep eluded me again, although there was no sign of the malady which had driven me to Sound Therapy. The cure was effective, but I mourned the loss of the beneficial side effects. For that I would have traded the cure in a twinkling.

I tried to cheer myself by going to some parties, now being normal, audiometrically speaking. Though I could stand the sound of voices, I remembered that I couldn't stand parties. I walked the fields, humming desperately. The humming technique I'd been taught was the one scrap of self-help possible. I hummed until the birds all fled from that part of Quebec! It helped a little, but without the high frequencies to back it up I was humming in the dark.

Writer's block struck again, and I was devastated. But there was something I could do for this. I developed a pattern: whenever I was seriously stuck I would phone Montreal and make an appointment for one Sound Therapy session. The three hours of listening never failed to get my inspiration flowing.

Evidently I was tied for life to the Montreal area, or maybe Toronto, where I understood there was one other sound therapist practising.

Life is cruel, and circumstances conspired to move me two years later to the Saskatchewan prairie. Settled in a tiny, charming old farmhouse in the Minichinas Hills, I knew it was the perfect place for me to live and write. Yet the real place of writing was in my head, and I would cheerfully have camped at the intersection of Peel and Ste. Catherine Streets if I could have had again the limitless vitality, the calm and drugless high that brought my inspiration to me like Joan's angel voices on the wind.

Two years passed, and ever my mind strained eastward. Running like an underground river through my thoughts were plans and schemes for getting more Sound Therapy. I was on the point more than once of applying as Writer-in-Residence at Montreal's Concordia University, a mad idea as I scarcely take up residence even in my own house but have to be always in the fresh air, doing my writing under the sky.

Sound Therapy at St Peter's Abbey, Muenster

Some people have a vivid, lifelong, shining memory of the moment when they were proposed to; or informed that they had won the Irish sweepstake; or received the inspiration for a great invention. I will carry a vivid, lifelong shining memory of the moment, one evening in my prairie farmhouse, when my dinner guest, Russ Powell, idly said:

"Oh, you know St. Peter's Abbey up at Muenster?" (I didn't know it. I just knew Muenster on the map.) "I have a relative by marriage there," he continued, "a monk named Father Lawrence —"

I stifled a yawn.

"— and he's working with the same therapy you took in Montreal."

"*What?*" I sprang up, toppling my chair. Russ looked a little alarmed. "Sound Therapy?"

"Yes," he said. "I went up last week and he demonstrated the listening test for me. They're using the therapy with the pre-vocation students at St. Peter's College there."

Muenster? *Muenster?* Could it be possible? Russ described the listening test and the electronic set-up. There was no doubt: it was the same. On the thousands of miles of prairie, I had landed blind, forty-eight miles from the kingdom.

Next morning at the crack of dawn I phoned St. Peter's, and of course found people up. Father Lawrence listened to my incoherent plea, and invited me to supper at the Abbey. There, in impeccably kept grounds and buildings, I found an alive brotherhood of educators, farmers and innovators. Father Lawrence DeMong was a warm, dynamic person, a practical visionary who had introduced Sound Therapy into the school more than two years before. It was

51

already here, I realized, when I was drawn across the country by what? That force which goes by many names.

He said: "I believe that Religious Houses like ours should be crossing new frontiers. Here's a new frontier which is really exciting but is not being crossed very rapidly. That's why we as an Abbey took this initiative."

Initiative didn't stop there. At supper I met Brother Oswald, who was into health foods and brought all his own makings to meals – raw vegetables, sunflower seeds, tofu, brown bread, herbal tea. He also practised Iridology and treated his brethren with a few other way-out healing techniques. They themselves didn't bother with the Sound Therapy, however. The listening took too much time and they were busy men.

After the meal Father Lawrence escorted me to the College wing where the listening lab was located. And there it was – the self-same array of intricate machines, all twenty thousand dollars worth. Twice: for there were two listening rooms side by side, each with its Electronic Ear and reel-to-reels and all the supporting gadgets.

My head still hadn't caught up with my feet, which had transported me as in a dream to this monastery in the middle of nowhere, which I found equipped with the very latest in electronic wizardry, leading the way toward new heights in education, healing and personal development. I couldn't quite grasp what this bearded priest in his blue jeans and sneakers was telling me. I thought he said I could come and listen just as much as I wanted to. Was it possible that he could give up all that time for my treatment? And I wondered if I could afford it. I inquired about the fee. He waved my question away with a smile.

"I'll give you a key to the listening room," he said. "You can come and listen any hour of the day or night."

Did that mean he intended to turn up at those times to operate the machinery?

"The listening rooms are in use during school hours, but come as early as you'd like in the mornings or you may prefer the evening. Stay all night if you want." He gestured to the sofas in the room. "Would you like to start immediately?"

"But what about my listening program?" I ventured to ask. Surely he had to work that out first.

"There are the tapes." He indicated a shelf lined with reel boxes. "They're all labelled. The 8,000 hertz gives the quickest recharge, but you can vary them for interest. Just help yourself."

I broke in politely. "Who's going to work the equipment, Father?"

"You are."

"Me?"

"I'll teach you right now," he said briskly. "I have a few minutes before prayers."

Learning to use the equipment

With an eye on his wristwatch, he flicked on the machines, and taking it for granted that I could understand plain English, said: "You adjust the intensity with this Gate – the Recorder lever has the same effect so you can use a combination of the two to throw the light from red to green, and the oftener you switch them the better. These dials control lateralization; you might want your right ear dominance to start at five and ten and work up to one and ten. Don't rush it. This is Volume, this is Power, be sure to turn it off when you leave."

"Do I have to press Stop?" I asked.

"No, it stops automatically." That was something anyway.

He selected one of the tapes at random and threaded it swiftly and deftly onto the reel. I think he had the impression he was showing me how. In the end I learned the whole business the way I learned to drive: got going with the thing and worked it out.

But I asked him now: "How will I know which tape to play first?"

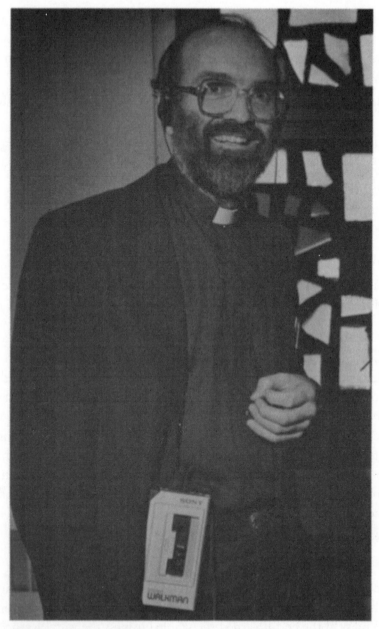

Father Lawrence DeMong was responsible for introducing the listening therapy at St Peter's

"The sequence makes no difference at all. I'll get your key now." He started for the door.

"But – but," I stammered, "What if I overdo it?"

"You can't overdo it. There's no way this sound can harm you. The more listening you do, the better. Some have listened for eight hours a day and it did them nothing but good." He went bounding off down the hall.

I looked at the Electronic Ear and it blinked its lights at me. Was this man actually going to leave us alone together?

Father hurried back in and handed me the key. "Sorry to run off. Happy listening!" he said, and rushed off to pray. I stood there with the key in my hand, the perfect symbol. It was the key to the kingdom.

But there was work ahead. First I sat down to listen to the tape that was already running on the reel. I was curious to hear what music they played here. I put on the headphones and to my amazement recognized the identical recording that had formed part of my therapy in Montreal. I wondered if the others were the same, though my curiosity was not satisfied quickly. It took me hours to get through another couple of half hour tapes. Yet I made progress. For instance, after a reel had fallen off the deck a few times and rolled across the floor with me crawling after it, I figured out the purpose of the little knob that holds it on.

And each tape I heard was a duplicate of those which I had thought designed for my particular hearing problem. In Montreal I had had the clear impression that the music and the order of the music were part of a personalized program. Here, as the guest of St. Peter's, I was invited to help myself. There hadn't even been any talk of a listening test – though they had the testing device, because there it was over in the corner.

I had enough to figure out for one night, so I let that one go.

By the time I turned everything off and locked the door the Abbey was silent and dark, with low lights in the corridors to guide me out. The outer doors were unlocked and unattended, with only the ancient trees standing guard. The moon spread its light over the stately grounds and gardens, and as I walked to my car I thought of what they said, people like these, about the answer to prayer – even if they had to run for it, as a result of setting someone on the path.

I rose before five the next morning in order to get to the Abbey by six o'clock. That way I could have three hours' listening before school started. I couldn't be sure it was really true until I fitted the key in the lock and found that it turned, admitting me to the room that was to become my second home. It was a large room, full of light, with a reclining chair and several couches. Tall windows gave a view of prairie sky, and below, the vast and perfect lawns. This time I omitted the sewing. I brought the tea and my writing pad. I brought my hopes... and they promised to be fulfilled. By nine o'clock the subtle dynamo was again whirring in my brain, though it would take a week to return to its former strength. I thought of the way people kiss the earth when they return to their native land after exile. I could have kissed the hardwood floor.

Better not, for the students were traipsing in, four or five big lads, casting curious looks at me in my headphones. Father Lawrence had said I might stay and share the facilities with them whenever I wished, as there were plenty of headphones, with small Volume/ Balance boxes on the floor to plug them into. At a later date he told me it did the kids good to see that someone would come in here and listen to this stuff of her own free will. For them it was compulsory, of course, since this was school. Compulsory or voluntary, it worked the same. I watched, marvelling, as they collected their headphones from the shelves and plugged them in and stretched out on the couches. If school had been like this for me, what might I not have amounted to by now?

I offered to let them change the tape I was playing if they wanted another. They said that was okay, it didn't matter, and plonked on their headphones and went to sleep.

The tapes and their special filtering

It was clicking into place for me. It really didn't make any difference which tape you listened to or what order you played them in. I had discovered that this entire set of tapes was identical to the ones I'd heard in Montreal, and was to find out that indeed the master tapes were made by Dr. Tomatis in Paris and purchased by the therapists, who then made their own copies. The therapeutic value was not in the assortment or the sequence, but in the filtering and Electronic Ear effect. The high frequency was imprinted on every tape and played to the patient through the Electronic Ear. You could have taken any one of them and benefited to the full by playing it often enough. The only trouble was that you'd tire of it, and that was the reason for the variety of music.

There was also a variation in the degree of filtering. One half hour tape began at normal and was gradually filtered up to 8,000 Hz. The next to be played was 8,000 Hz from start to finish. A third began at 8,000 and slowly descended to normal. That was the listening program. There was no deception in calling it that; it's just that the program was the same here as it had been in Montreal and came down to the fact that all you have to do is play the music. After a certain length of time the brain becomes harmonized and energized. It then begins giving the right signals to the rest of the system, and ease replaces disease.

Father Lawrence acknowledged that that's what it boiled down to. Yet he claimed it was useful to give the students the listening test; it provided an accurate diagnosis, and the students' progress could then be checked.

A case in point: before the school term ended I was invited to address the English class. I read from one of my plays, and afterwards a girl came up to me and expressed her appreciation. She was quite eloquent. When she had moved on, Sister Miriam Spenrath, her English teacher, said to me: "One year ago that girl had such a speech defect that you could hardly understand her. She's been on the Sound Therapy program, listening an hour a day for one year. Her latest listening test showed an eighty percent improvement."

I hadn't noticed any flaw in the girl's speech at all. I wondered why they needed a machine to measure her improvement and couldn't just measure it by the girl. But that's science for you.

At the same time I could understand why the therapy had to be framed into a structure for treating the public. It has been established that the average time required for the effect to begin is 100 to 200 hours. Therefore my initial six weeks, at fifteen hours a week, was pretty close and fulfilled its claim by healing my intolerance to cross-vibrations of sound. If the six weeks was not long enough to lock in the accompanying gift of radiant energy, well, that was never presented as a feature of the therapy. It was simply a bonus which came along for a time, and which I wanted to grasp and hang onto for life.

Beneficial side-effects of long-term listening

Now the question arose – was it possible to make permanent connection with that great reservoir of energy, to which we ordinarily have such a clogged pipeline? As far as I could discover, no-one had ever listened long enough to find out. Unless you were really suffering, the therapy was too great a sacrifice in time. No-one wanted to sit hour after hour, helplessly plugged in, while life with its demands clamoured outside the door. Even Father Lawrence who directed the program said he sat down in the lab and listened only when desperately tired or preparing for some test of endurance.

Well, if that was the only problem, I was going to make myself a test case. I settled into a routine which I was determined to stick to for as long as it took. Rising at four a.m. every day, I left the house at five, drove into the Abbey grounds at six, and listened for three hours alone with my writing. I got a lot of work done and started to really enjoy the technical business of manipulating the tapes and reels. Monitoring the Electronic Ear myself gave a sense of direct contact, of being in touch, like running my own life instead of having it controlled from the next room. I was getting the hang of this fabulous equipment, and was still amazed that anyone would leave me alone with it. There were dozens of dials and levers that had to do with the recording process; these I eyed with fear and was careful not to touch.

I put on the tape with the sibilant sounds and had a go at the microphone; also the Gregorian chant. The voice recharge in combination with the ear was considered extremely valuable, and I could feel the effect immediately. But the mike was a hassle, and I decided to do my singing on the prairie, where I walked miles every day anyway. I hit on the idea of plugging my ears with cotton for return resonance and felt a good effect from it. The reason the humming worked for me, where it hadn't on my farm walks in Quebec, was that now I had the boost of the daily high frequencies. I would also find with time that I could sing in tune, as I never could before.

After about a week I was back to the energy level of the therapy days in Montreal. Because of that groundwork, the whole process was speeded up this time. Around the middle of the week I again passed through the sluggish sea of tiredness, but left it behind after a day or two. Despite the four a.m. rising I rode high on energy all day and once more was able to cut out the hour's rest I'd always needed after lunch. Time was very precious to me and I had always resented the time given for sleep – that daytime hour especially. I did start to fade out after supper and began to wish I lived next door to the Abbey, for I knew that half an hour's listening would set me up again for the evening.

Sound Therapy on the Walkman™

The two hours a day I had to spend on the road travelling to and from the monastery were quite a loss, but I tried not to worry about that. The gains were worth it. I whiled away the journey listening to symphonies on my Sony Walkman™, a new acquisition which I treasured above all things. Father Lawrence spotted it one day

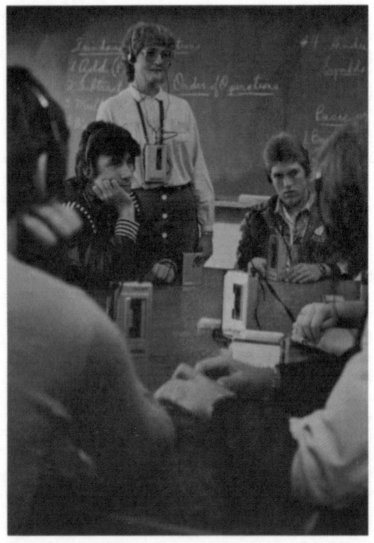

Sister Miriam Spenrath and her students at St Peter's College listen in class and, at the very least, are much less frazzled at the end of the day than many teachers and pupils

and was immediately interested. This was before everybody and his brother had one, and the marvel of it was still new. Actually, he was interested in getting one for his brother, who had a birthday coming up. Always conscious of frequencies, he asked me what the frequency response was. As if I would know! I looked it up in the booklet that night, and next morning I told him. It was 16,000 hertz.

"Sixteen thousand!" he exclaimed. "Why, it's high enough for you to do your therapy on the Walkman™."

We were standing at dead centre of the main lobby, in a pool of sunlight which came pouring down from a high window. He was wearing his black robes and beyond him the sun caught the switchboard, the girl dressed in pink behind the glass, sparkling like a fish in tropical waters. The details are etched on my memory, because it was another of those moments that cast their aura over the whole of life.

"Buy some metal cassettes," he went on briskly. "Half a dozen should do. Bring them with you tomorrow. I'll set up a cassette deck in the lab and take the day off and we'll record the whole program for you." He said that while their equipment ran to 20,000 hertz, it took a very sensitive ear to hear 16,000. And he knew that the cheap imitations of the Walkman™ didn't approach that level. It would seem that with a little extra listening to the cassettes, the Sony should yield the full therapy effect.

I drove home with my tires one foot off the road. That afternoon I went shopping for metal cassettes. When I discovered the price I hardly flinched. At the cost of the formal Tomatis therapy per hour, I would pay as much to listen for that length of time just once.

Next day the listening lab was closed to the students. Some of them listened in the other listening room, while the remainder spent the time cleaning the schoolrooms and seemed to much prefer it. Father Lawrence was expert at recording, bringing into action some more of the mysterious lights and buttons. Completely awed I watched him juggling wires, twirling knobs and dials and monitoring the dance of the arrows. I thought again how far the Church had come. Time was, he'd have been burned at the stake for this.

At the end of the afternoon he placed the six cassettes in my hands and said, "We'll miss you, but now you can do all your listening at home."

So now the prayer was fully answered and there was nothing more to do.

(Oh no?)

Listening to Sound Therapy in public

It happened that the next day I couldn't do my listening at home, for it was shopping day, the occasion of the week that always filled me with dread. Though a mixture of voices could now be tolerated, I remained atmosphere-sensitive and couldn't stand the din of traffic or the psychically crushing environment of supermarkets and shopping malls. My daughter did the driving, which helped; and she lugged everything around and made decisions after my mind was blown. This was not the daughter who had introduced me to Sound Therapy, but my youngest, Felicity, whom I now lived with in a delightful partnership not in the least marred by her total indifference to the discovery which had changed my life. She loved rock (which accounted for us long ago introducing headphones into the house), and thought Tomatis an old fogey who just didn't know real music when he heard it.

Well, if I couldn't listen to my new therapy cassettes at home, at least I could take them with me. I played the music throughout the forty minute drive to Saskatoon, and the half hour finding a place to park, with the volume set low so that we could talk. Then I kept it on, the Walkman™ tucked in my shoulder bag, as we went around the stores.

Soon an amazing thing became apparent. It was as though I walked on a battlefield with a shield held before me and my head protected by armour. The noise was still there; my mind registered the fact like information of no particular significance. If there were cross-currents of psychic agitation, they found in my immediate atmosphere a wall of harmony that could not be breached.

After an hour or two, when I would normally have been a wreck, I was discovering that shopping could be fun. I wanted to investigate the sales. But we didn't have time, because it was turning into "one of those days." As chance would have it – or was it fateful design? – our ancient Volvo broke down three (3) times in traffic, making us the focus of all eyes as we waited for the mechanic. I drew some particularly strange looks, sitting there under a mantle of tranquillity with my headphones on, and being somewhat beyond the age of the average music addict. The spectators would have been even more surprised if they could have heard what I was hearing.

Sharing the therapy around

The thought that other people might hear it one day did not flower just then, but the seed may have stirred in the serene depths of my mind. It was the next morning as I walked out on the prairie with my Walkman™, listening to the sweet high frequencies for the first time beneath the open sky, that the idea sprang up full blown. This gift which had landed in my lap was surely not intended for me alone – or for the few who already knew of it. Presently it was limited to the elect, to those who lived in Toronto or Montreal, and could pay the price – most especially the three hours a day sitting immobilized. Those had to be people in real trouble. But everybody is in a little bit of trouble. Who doesn't need more energy, more time, more peace of mind?

A lot of people already owned a Walkman™. Even if they had to buy one … I placed it against the alternative, which is to own the original equipment, at 20,000 Hz and $20,000. That's a dollar a hertz. The Sony Walkman™ at 16,000 Hz and a price of, let's say, a hundred dollars (some models are less, some more) works out to 1/160th of the cost. Judging by my experience in town the previous day, the lower frequency response didn't make that much difference. And once people had the therapy cassettes, they could also play them on their home tape decks, many at 18,000 to 20,000 Hz.

And who was going to get this going? I looked up at the vast prairie sky and knew I was elected. I stumbled into a gopher hole, which provided perspective and encouraged me to sit down and think about the whole thing.

I would have to research the subject, write about it, talk a lot, and experiment with the cassettes to see if they would work as well as the standard therapy. This meant getting some cassettes in circulation. I couldn't very well copy the Tomatis tapes and hand them out, so would have to produce my own. That meant making master tapes.

That meant finding out how the music was filtered – and doing it myself. The therapists obtained the music already filtered, and simply ran it through the Electronic Ear directly to the patient. I would have to filter the music and record it in the same process with the Electronic Ear.

Ye gods, I'd have to understand the Electronic Ear! But why had I been trying so hard to shake my brain awake, if it wasn't to understand more, learn more, do more with my life? If this was a little more than I'd bargained for, maybe I was forgetting the Bargainer at the other end of the deal.

I drove up to St. Peter's that afternoon and explained why I was back so soon. I wanted to go about introducing Sound Therapy, economy style, mobile and self-directed, to a larger public. The monks accepted the idea as logical, practical, and therefore quite likely inspired. I was offered the full use of their facilities, and all the help I needed. It was a good thing they threw in the second part of the offer.

Learning how to filter the music

I mentioned that I didn't even know how the music was filtered. They informed me that it was done with two filtering machines, and they already possessed these at the Abbey, for the filtering of mothers' voices. (More about that later.)

"They're a bit complicated," Father Lawrence said cheerfully.

A bit? The moment I came face to face with those filters my heart failed me. The monks gathered round. "You can do it," they said.

There was a sound expert in the Order, a young brother with the patience of Job, and he was assigned to instruct me in the Catechism of Electronics.

And bit by bit the mysterious became knowable, the complex yielded its secrets and stood revealed as simple. Well anyway, possible. I learned how to record the music from records onto reels, filtering the low frequencies out imperceptibly, so that the ear doesn't know what's happening and adjusts painlessly to the high sounds that are ambrosia for the brain. At the same time it was being recorded through the Electronic Ear. But when transferred from reels to cassettes, there were problems of distortion in the high frequencies.

How to solve it? That's what I had to figure out. Everyone was very busy around there, and I couldn't forever be pressing the button to central switchboard – the one I used the most – and calling for Brother William. It was summer; school was out and the listening lab, now converted to recording room, was mine. Along with the original pieces of equipment there were now two cassette decks, a turntable, amplifier, and the two big black frequency equalizers with their special filter adaptations. To this I added a few electric devices of a personal sort: my typewriter, a kettle for my tea, a negative ion generator (we won't get into that right now) and a lamp on a long cord for better scrutiny of the numbered levers in the midnight hours. I'm surprised I didn't blow the whole monastery into eternal darkness. There were so many wires that strangers venturing in might have thought they were in a den of snakes. I learned to make my way through them, trailing more wires from my ears, and only occasionally getting so tangled up I resorted to prayer – or words of that nature.

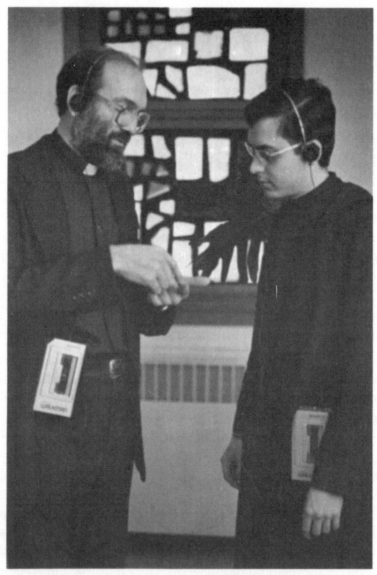

The twentieth century in the Abbey. Father Lawrence, with organist and electronics expert Brother William Thurmeier

There wasn't much danger of strangers wanting to come in. All that summer, visitors passing the open door stopped and froze. The place looked more as though it belonged to Buck Rogers than to God. But God is showing His scientific streak these days, and if some of it falls on His shadow side, all the more reason to catch what is thrown with the other hand and run with it.

I was experimenting and learning at the same time, working every day and late into the nights. My learning was from the ground up, as I reached for the stars. The combining of filtered music with the Electronic Ear in a single process presented problems which no-one had ever encountered before. Anyone with real experience at recording would not have tried. Here was where complete ignorance had the advantage. I didn't know it couldn't work, so I stumbled blindly along seeking answers. Not quite blindly: I had tips from the monks as they poked their heads in from time to time to see how I was getting on. Some ventured in further and asked if they might listen; they had always wondered what this Sound Therapy was all about.

Friends and advisers

An important adviser was Father Andrew, principal of the College. He was knowledgeable about music and familiar with the equipment. Dropping in one day he casually offered a piece of counsel which proved to be crucial – something I wouldn't have hit on in a thousand years.

I made many friends. Brother Oswald, quick to spot another health freak, stopped by in stray moments to talk about healing systems. He knew them all. I learned quite a bit about Iridology. Iridology isn't much known yet in the outer world, so no-one had better try telling me that the monastic life means withdrawal from the business of human progress. It seemed to me a truth that you have to step back in order to get a broader and more selective view.

Father Lawrence was always around in the background. As the Abbey's sound therapist he had a few summer patients coming in from outside. He used the equipment in the next room, as I had this one tied up, and conducted the treatment just as he had with me: he showed them how to work everything, then left them to it. He still couldn't spare the time to do any listening himself. One of his patients was Sister Anne Honig from Edmonton, who was spending her vacation at the Abbey, having chosen it for its Sound Therapy facility. She was one of the few visitors who wasn't afraid to ask me what I was doing. We shared midnight tea and she tried out some of my cassettes. A few of the monks were testing them for me too, using my Walkman™. I often lent it out for the day and sometimes had trouble finding it when I wanted to go home. I never travelled without it.

Driving home at night or in the very early mornings, I listened to the cassettes I'd made that day to check them out. This was after listening to high frequencies for eight or ten hours at a stretch. When I saw the sky shimmering with Northern lights I thought possibly it was coming out of my head. Yet despite this perpetual high, sleep came to me as to a child. I found it true that as the energy rises the relaxation deepens, and the expansion is an indication of expanding life.

The word spreads

It started happening that I would walk into the recording room and run into one monk or another, apologizing to me for using the space, but as everything was set up and adjusted he thought he'd just turn out a few cassettes of his own. Father Lawrence had persuaded the Muenster Elks, a wide awake, forward-looking group, to donate a number of Walkman™s, and he had gone out and bought a hundred metal tapes. He explained to me that you saved money buying in quantity, though I already knew that argument well.

So at last this marvellous vitalizing sound that he had brought to the Abbey was accessible to him; he had the time to listen – because it didn't take any. Parish priest, educator, therapist, he kept up with it all as he strode around with his headphones on and his Walkman™

in the pocket of his robe. It was a boon, another father told me, because he hadn't been sleeping well before he started this, and their early rising applied whether they slept or not.

Brother William, my mentor, was off for a year's study at a seminary in the States, and cassette players were not allowed. He obtained special permission to bring his Sony Walkman™ and the therapy cassettes, as an aid to study. Sister Anne, whose therapy had been doing so much good she dreaded leaving it, headed back to Edmonton with a Walkman™ and six-pack of cassettes.

By the end of the summer, half a dozen monks, a handful of nuns and the janitor were walking around St. Peter's with headphones on. Transferred to Ottawa, Father Lawrence made the drive alone at the wheel with a minimum of sleep (apart from a few breaks for snoozes), listening to the therapy cassettes all the way.

Word travelled to the sisters at the Ursuline Convent of Bruno not far away. Two of their elderly sisters were suffering from Alzheimer's disease, that dread deterioration of the brain for which there is no cure. Might the Sound Therapy help? They bought four Walkman™s and a collection of cassettes. Six weeks later the nursing staff reported that the two sisters with Alzheimer's were "greatly improved – more settled, less hyper and enjoying the music recreationally."

The word from Ottawa was that Father Lawrence wasn't listening much any more, because every time he met a kid with severe problems he gave away his whole set-up.

An unlikely technical adviser

Early in the fall the decision was made at St. Peter's College to introduce the Walkman™ system in the classrooms so that the students could listen as they worked. More cassettes would have to be made. But the equipment in the recording room was all disassembled. Brother William had gone; Father Lawrence had gone. Many of the monks knew how to handle run-of-the-mill recording, but this meant getting into the really complicated stuff.

So guess who was called in to advise?

I'd been so busy through the summer that a certain point had escaped my attention. It was one afternoon as I sat deeply concentrated, monitoring four machines at once, that it hit me. This was the same person who once couldn't get along with a toaster!

What had caused the transformation? It was the sound itself, opening my mind to capacities that had been slumbering, snoring in fact, so deep asleep they would have moved without stirring into the grave.

And what else was sleeping there, and sleeps in everyone? We're told that even geniuses use only ten percent of their brain. Within his own operative ten percent one genius named Tomatis had found a way for us to begin the trek into the limitless potential of the rest.

Oh and by the way, you can fold all the paper bags you want while I'm around, as long as I get my headphones on first!

Chapter Three

The Tomatis Effect

> **"** *We are creatures of sound. We live in it and it lives in us.* **"**
> *But this is a fact we have forgotten, just as the fish forgets*
> *that it lives in water.*
>
> Dr. Alfred Tomatis

Tomatis was intrigued by work done with unborn birds showing how they recognize the voices of their mothers. This statement captured him: "The eggs of song birds hatched under silent foster mothers produce songless young."

Was it possible that a similar phenomenon might occur in utero between the human mother and child? Hypothesizing that at some time in prenatal life, the foetus might be able to hear the sounds produced by the mother's voice, Dr. Tomatis decided to explore what he thought the intra-uterine world might sound like.

The mother's voice

He wrapped a microphone and speaker in a thin rubber membrane and immersed them in water. The speaker was connected to a tape of one of his client's voices. The microphone was connected to another tape recorder, thus registering the sound from the speaker when passed through water. The sound was extraordinary. It reminded him of a deep African night beside the river, containing unusually high frequencies, mostly above 8,000 Hz. When tested on patients, listening to their mothers' voices recorded through layers of water, the foundation was laid for new research into foetal life. Since then it has been proven that the foetus does hear. Its ear is functional from the fourth month;[10] and Tomatis suggests that from that time it hears the mother's voice and registers all the sounds of her vegetative life.[11]

Early in his experiments, Tomatis had referred to him a fourteen-year-old autistic child, who had apparently cut himself off from communication at the age of four. A filtered recording was made of the mother's voice and played to the child. The results were dramatic: the boy turned off the lights in the room, curled up on his mother's lap in a foetal position and sucked his thumb throughout the session. Tomatis gradually reduced the filtering until the voice was like normal air-conducted sound. As the filtering was reduced the boy began to babble like a ten-month-old child. Thus was born the term Sonic Birth, the passage from audition in liquidian milieu to audition in aerial milieu, which is the central image and concept of the Tomatis Sound Therapy. (We aren't told what happened to that particular autistic child, but others appear to have been aided by the filtered sounds.)

Tomatis says: "By means of filtered sounds through the medium of a memorized ancient audition, we arouse the awakening of the most archaic relationship desired: the relationship with the mother. There is no doubt possible. It shall be found in utero. In order to awaken this same process, we provoke a revival of this very first audition."

The result of this work is an effective treatment for children with problems of learning, communication and perception. The therapist records the mother's voice, filtered to high frequency, reading a story which the child will like. This is then relayed to the child through the Electronic Ear.[12]

---

10 Birnholz J.C. et al. "The development of human fetal hearing", *Science* (1983), 222. 516-518.
11 Tomatis, A.A., *The Conscious Ear*, Station Hill Press, New York, 1991.
12 Gilmor, T.M. Madaule, P. & Thompson, B.M. (eds) *About The Tomatis Method*, the Listening Centre Press, Toronto, 1989.

A therapist says: "One would have to be present at these unforgett-able sessions in order to fully grasp the impact of such a venture. Hearing the filtered maternal voice, the child changes his relationship with the mother; he becomes more affectionate and closer to her, much to her great satisfaction, for she feels more loved and needed. As the sessions progress there is a change in the child's behaviour, both at home and at school. The parents tell us that their child is more present, that he listens better, he understands better what is said to him, he concentrates more easily and takes a greater part in the life of the home. Because he begins to be able to analyze the sound messages that come his way, the universe becomes more comprehensible to him. We see here the importance of the discriminating power of the ear. From here on, one may consider specific teaching for such a child and expect the integration of such notions as rules of grammar. He is then able to learn in half an hour what his mother or his teacher had tried for several years to make him learn."

Tomatis does say that when it is impossible to record the mother's voice, one may simply proceed with the filtered music training.

Portable Sound Therapy benefits children

A variety of problems have yielded to the portable therapy in the short while it has been in use; and its usage increases as it is shown to be of value to the troubled and the healthy alike. Sister Miriam of St. Peter's tells of dining with a family who provided Walkmans™ and therapy cassettes for each of their three children. The children come in from playing and reach for the headphones instead of turning on the television. They enjoy the filtered music, as most children will if it isn't forced on them. In this instance it is used as prevention rather than cure.

Play itself is an important element of protection against disorders. Research has shown that cortical and sub-cortical activities must be in balance for keeping the organism stable.[13] Children receive an

---

13 Wenner, M., "The Serious Need for Play." *Scientific American Mind*, 39, Feb 2009.

overdose of cortical burdening, because they have little free time and increasing school loads. School demands cortical activity for nine-tenths of the time spent there. It's not natural for children to subordinate their sub-cortical activity to cortical control for long hours of the day. For the growing child the one-sided overburdening of the cortex may cause irreparable damage. The increase of childhood hypertensions and neuroses give warning about the need for much more recreation and freedom.

The reading disability known as dyslexia has become a concern in the last few decades. The problem was hardly known in the last generation. Today it seems much more prevalent and is said to affect from five to 17 percent of school-aged children, with as many as 40 percent of the entire population reading below grade level.[14] The dyslexic child is one who has reading difficulties that are incompatible with his or her intellectual potential. Such children are usually considered to be slow learners, and are perhaps even labelled stupid or retarded. Bright dyslexic children can be indistinguishable from the less gifted normal children: they don't like school, they hate learning, they can't concentrate, they refuse to exert an effort. If their condition is not addressed they may be deprived of the opportunity measure up to their full potential in life.

Tomatis has successfully treated more than 12,000 dyslexics in centres which he has established in Europe and Africa. He says: "We read with our ears." A child may be dyslexic before ever encountering the written word. Reading is not a mechanical process of decoding symbols. Children are not naming letters when they read, but rather are listening to their own voice, whether reading silently or aloud. They are also listening to what the author has to say. Reading is a form of communication, and the auditory processing required for listening is one of the foundations of reading.[15]

Listening is not the same as hearing. Listening is a voluntary act. A

14 Shaywitz, S.E. and Shaywitz, "The Neurobiology of Reading and Dyslexia" *Focus on Basics,* National Center for the Study of Adult Learning and Literacy, Volume 5, Issue A August 2001. Reference added 2009.

15 Tomatis, A. A. *The Ear and Language.* Moulin. Ontario, 1996.

lack of desire to communicate causes many children with perfectly acute hearing to shut off their ears to the spoken word. A mother says: "If I talk to my son in a normal voice he doesn't hear. But when I repeat the words in a low booming voice, he looks up right away."

The child has deafened himself in the high frequencies. This we have all done in varying degrees and for reasons which are many and individual. It starts at the very beginning of life. Tomatis says that on the tenth day after birth, from the moment when the Eustachian tube empties its liquid, the infant becomes plunged into sonoric darkness, which prevents it from hearing the elevated frequencies that it heard during its foetal life. It doesn't yet know how to tense its musculature (the tympanus) in the air medium to recover its perception of the very high frequencies.[16] The ear will have to carry on the work of accommodation and concentration for many years in order to retrieve the high levels needed for communication. In many instances the child falls short of this recovery. This is one reason why wise and informed child-care is so vital in the early years. The human species is characterized by the elasticity of the central nervous system, and children are born with a perception of frequency ranging from 16 cycles to about 20,000 or more. This is the range of sound perception that is available to them. But in their life experience they will settle down to cater to those frequencies which they find useful or indispensable to their immediate environment. Although possessing a wide range 'keyboard' of the inner ear, they do not necessarily use it all; by using only what is useful for them they restrict their range.

Tuning in or tuning out

One important function of the ear is to suppress visceral or self-produced sounds so that attention can be paid to external sounds. The tympanus is either relaxed and deaf to external stimuli, or properly tensed to tune in to the outside input. In children whose

---

16 Ibid.

inner needs are not met, their attention will remain attached to the internal world of the viscera, and interest in the outside world will be hampered. Outside sounds, such as the spoken word, will have an emotional connotation for the child that may well be quite separate from the meaning of the words themselves. The speaker will be perceived as reassuring or threatening. The child will respond by tuning the person in or out, according to the affective message the voice holds. In negative situations the child will shut off the ear to the analysis and discrimination of speech sounds, being either too frightened by the message that is conveyed or too preoccupied with the inner visceral sounds. Hearing, therefore, becomes a matter not simply of sound, but of the way in which the message inherent in the sound is interpreted by the listener.

Children learn to tune out their parents, and when they get to school they begin tuning out the teacher by the same process. Selectivity, meaning the ability to select from the full range of sounds, is by then blocked, either on all frequencies, right and left, or on only one part of the sound scale for both ears, or for one ear only.

There is another way of withdrawing from auditory communication and from entering the world of grown-ups through language, Tomatis suggests, and that is by lowering the threshold of one's hearing to the point of apparent deafness. One of the standard complaints of parents and teachers is that so many children do not listen. The problem lies in a non-listening attitude. These children lack motivation and are unable to discriminate sounds. Another trick consists in shuffling the cards, to no longer know where sound comes from, to live in confusion. There is no earthly use in nagging such children to tidy up their rooms; that only adds to the chaos in their heads and aggravates their difficulty in spatialization.

Then there is the child who chooses to keep others at a distance by choosing the longer circuits, that is by borrowing the left auditory route. The left hemisphere of the brain is the centre of symbolic thought and language, and the right ear is the most direct route to this centre. For efficient analysis of language, the right ear must be the directing ear. The left ear has to use a longer, less efficient route, and when neither ear consistently leads we see the phenomenon of reversals. For example, in the word **saw**, if the 's' is 'heard' by the left ear and the 'w' is heard by the right, the 'w' will reach the left hemisphere before the 's' and the child will read **was**.

The importance of right ear dominance

In the treatment of dyslexia, then, not only is the filtered music used to open the ear to the full range of frequencies, but lateralization to the right is developed. This is done by continually feeding more sound into the right ear than the left. Dr. Tomatis found that when he put earphones on the children and increased the sound to the right ear, they spoke more eagerly, their reading ability improved, and their behaviour improved as well.

Tomatis's theory of auditory laterality, or the dominance of the right ear, was developed through intensive experiments with singers. It resulted in his First Law: the voice contains only what the ear hears; or, more scientifically: the larynx emits only the harmonics that the ear can hear.

He had his subjects sing and monitor themselves with both ears through headphones, while he made a sonogram which pictured a normal, well timbred, sonorous voice. Next, Tomatis 'tuned out' the right ear electronically (by leaving it out of the circuit) thus forcing the subjects to listen and monitor themselves through the left ear. The subsequent diagram showed the disappearance of an entire series of harmonics. At the same time the singers found themselves slowing down; they noted that they were tired; they felt oppressed and had trouble singing in tune. Next, the singers monitored themselves with the right ear, that is they blocked out the sound of the left as it returned to them through the earphones. The diagram which resulted showed an impressive display of harmonics, even greater in content than the one where the self-monitoring was done through both ears. The subjects said that they found it very pleasant to sing in this way, and they could do it with greater facility than usual. They felt light and had a sense of well-being; the oppressed feeling had disappeared. The improvement in the voice, both in timbre and pitch, was obvious to the experimenter's ears.

Tomatis states categorically that great voices, sung or spoken, are the voices directed and controlled by the right ear and never by the left.

The same experiment performed with actors showed that speaking while monitoring with the left ear caused difficulties with timbre, concentration, attention, expression of thoughts, and finally a great tendency to fatigue. Further investigation proved conclusively that deficiencies of the voice are related to deficiencies of the ear.[17] By systematically comparing the hearing and speech curves of subjects suffering from scotomas (hearing loss at a particular frequency), Tomatis was able to show that there is an exact and total correspondence for all frequencies shown on the audiogram (the sounds heard) and on the phonogram (the sounds emitted.) Tomatis observed that when, through training with Sound Therapy, the frequencies that have been lost were restored to the ear, those frequencies were instantaneously and unconsciously restored to the voice.[18]

Thus he earned the profound gratitude of many singers and actors. The enhancement of range and harmonics in the voice is also a great boon to teachers – and those who have to listen to them. In fact, as we speak to each other, we are exerting an immense influence over others and upon ourselves. When we speak we use an instrument which surrounds us – the air. The aerial medium is full of life; all the molecules which surround us have a speed, called relative mean speed, and this is a permanent excitation, a pressure affecting our entire body. The instant we speak or hear a sound, the air changes in its state of pressure; it becomes physically modified and begins to caress the whole body, as when we are in the bath and agitate the water and the body feels it. Every time we speak, we flood our neurons, and, on the basis of acoustic pressure, we integrate all

---

17 Tomatis, A. A. *The Ear and Language.* Moulin. Ontario, 1996.
18 Ibid.

the information that we send. To speak and to speak well gives us enormous awareness of our body as a whole, and also affects the body of the listener. Nothing is as penetrating as someone else's voice. A voice either attacks or caresses the other's being. It enters through all the pores by pressure over the entire body, as well as through the apparatus of the ear.

Those who speak well have achieved what Tomatis calls right ear dominance. His experiments in laterality were not limited to the voice, but included virtuoso performers, especially violinists. The results were the same as with the singers. When forced to monitor themselves with the left ear, they lost their ability to play well and accurately. They were hampered in their movements, which stiffened and became slower. One said to Tomatis: "Not only am I hindered in my playing, but more than that, my fingers are paralyzed."

Sound Therapy for stuttering and speech difficulties

Such observations caused Tomatis to notice the delay in rhythm which led to stuttering, and he began working with stutterers. He says: "I had about 74 stutterers and I lived with them for a year. My biggest problem was not to start stuttering. All of the stutterers had trouble hearing from the right, and all of them, when I started them using the right ear alone, began to speak correctly." Later he used the same system in treating children with speech difficulties, and found that not only their speech but their behaviour changed; they became more dynamic, more open and eager to talk, and their parents reported that their reading had improved.

Dr E. Spirig of the Anvers Centre, Belgium, gives demonstrations of this at the Centre, using electronic equipment to produce the same reactions in volunteers chosen from among their visitors. He states: "By having volunteers read for a certain length of time while monitoring themselves with the *left* ear, we have been able to produce magnificent experimental dyslexics."

Listening difficulties and posture

Children with listening difficulties are often seen to have poor posture. These are helped both mentally and physically by the therapy, for the main nerves affected are the auditory nerve which dynamizes the cortex, and the vestibular nerve which determines posture.[19] The two nerves interact in a complementary way; each time the cortex is charged by picking up high frequency sounds through the ear, the vestibular nerve is influenced and improves the body schema.

Dr Spirig writes: "If we observe children who are retarded in language, or children who stutter, or are mentally defective, we find they have stooped or curved backs. It does little good to remind them a dozen times a day to stand up straight. These children receive too little charging of the cortex, too little stimulation of the vestibular nerve. They have the look of a beaten dog. Only an auditory re-education by means of the Electronic Ear will bring about a permanent change in their posture. They become vertical through language."

Similar work is being done with children who have cerebral palsy, who tend to have challenges with communication and emotional adjustment. Intensive training by means of the Electronic Ear enables new brain pathways to develop, opening new doors to potential and achievement.

The stimulation of the auditory pathways and resulting re-awakening of the desire to communicate, demonstrates again and again the degree to which deficiencies are related to blockages of listening. We live most of our lives unaware of these obstructions which impede our motivation and disrupt our communication with each other. Those who have not experienced the Sound Therapy listening cannot realize what they are missing by keeping their distortions. It is so easy to hear and to communicate once the ear is open to the external world, whereas it is so difficult to relate harmoniously to

---

19 Weeks, Bradford S., "The Therapeutic Effect of High Frequency Audition and its Role in Sacred Music". See Appendix. (Footnote added 2009)

the environment when one must constantly correct, on the cortical level, the distortions that complicate existence.

Tomatis on right and left-handedness

Whenever laterality is discussed, the question of left-handedness arises. In all civilizations, since earliest times, right-handedness has been the norm, with approximately ten percent of the population being left-handed.[20] According to Tomatis's theory of laterality, the right-handed person has more straightforward functional integration. Tomatis attributes laterality to the development of language, since deaf mutes are generally lacking in any noticeable laterality. "Language and the need to control it created the need to construct laterality," he writes.[21]

It's not that left-handed people are not as smart or as capable of achievement, but the same degree of achievement would seem to require more effort, due to their having to adapt to a right handed world. To see that life is harder for them, you only have to watch a lefty in the excruciating act of writing. I can say that, because I am one myself. The general coercion of my school days began with my being compelled to switch over from my left to my right – perhaps because I wrote my name, Pat, as Tap. The changeover may have been a good thing, though Tap Joudry on my books later in life might have been an eye-catcher and helped them sell! Psychologists later put a stop to the practice, claiming it would cause stuttering; although according to Tomatis, stuttering was more likely to result from leaving things as they were. At any rate, all my life since, I have written with my right hand and stubbornly done everything else with my left, and the only time I stutter is when the bank manager calls.

Tomatis has made a unique exploration of the complex relationship between handedness and ear dominance. To investigate this,

---

20 Tomatis, A. A. *The Ear and Language*. Moulin. Ontario, 1996. (Footnote added 2009)
21 Ibid. (Footnote added 2009)

he asked himself one day whether one might make lefties right-handed without letting them know, by working on their ear. He finally decided to take the step with one of his own children, three of whom were left-handed. He worked on his son's right ear, and at a certain point, spontaneously, the boy changed to the right hand. His efficiency and speed of learning also increased, and his speech became more controlled.

Tomatis says: "When I treat the right ear, it sometimes happens that the left-handed child starts mixing his handedness: he is hesitant. I encourage him by saying that he is not giving up his left hand, but that it has other tasks to perform. For a while he is disconcerted because his right hand is a clumsy instrument. But in a very short while it takes over, and there is no more conflict."

While this spontaneous change is sometimes seen in children who are still developing their laterality, this is not to say that for the majority of left handed listeners, Sound Therapy will influence them to change their dominant hand. It should be stressed that the aim of Sound Therapy is not to change handedness, but to change ear dominance to the right. Some have raised concerns about whether Sound Therapy is suitable for left-handers and should they reverse the headphones? The answer is that the headphones should be used as normal. Because the language seat is still in the left hemisphere for the great majority of left-handers,[22] right ear dominance is still appropriate. They do generally have a greater degree of ambidexterity than right-handers,[23] perhaps giving them access to a greater range of potential skills, and this added complexity of brain pathways may mean that the process of adaptation to Sound Therapy may be a little more convoluted and require more persistence.

Tomatis tells us also that laterality is sometimes quite fluid, and gives an example which occurred at an industrial depot, where he

---

22 Pujol, J., Deus, J. Losilla, J.M., and Capdevila, A., "Cerebral Lateralization of Language in Normal Left-handed People Studied by Functional MRI" *Neurology* 1999;52:1038 (Footnote added 2009)
23 Hardyk, C. and Petrinovich, L. F. "Left handedness," *Phsychological Bulletin,* Vol 84, No. 3, 1977. (Footnote added 2009)

was doing tests with workers' hearing. "At the depot the majority was right-handed. As the people work on jets they are engaged in precision work and subject to a high level of fatigue. On Monday morning they are all right-handed; Thursday and Friday evening, before they quit work, they are casualties of mixed laterality; they are neither right nor left-handed. At that point they are also hesitant to talk to anybody. They feel that their apparatus of feedback is not functioning properly. If one gave them a rifle for trial, I am sure they would not be able to aim at a target either. All their aiming potential has been damaged."

Such confusion of laterality, induced by stress, fades blissfully away as Sound Therapy's streamlined laterality, with a clear right-ear/left-brain language pattern becomes firmly established.

Chapter Four

Sleep

> ❝ *When I lay down to sleep, miraculously, I slept!* ❞
>
> Patricia Joudry

> ❝ *We are the music makers,* ❞
> *And we are the dreamers of dreams,*
> *Wandering by lone sea breakers,*
> *And sitting by desolate streams*
>
> A. O'Shaughnessy
> "The Music Maker"

Medical science showed little interest in sleep prior to the 1930s, leaving the subject to poets and dream interpreters who gave it their own mystical meanings. Then the EEG was invented, allowing scientists to use electrodes to measure brain waves.[24] This enabled the identification of several different levels of sleep. The main division is between REM, rapid eye movement or dreaming sleep, and NREM, non-rapid eye movement, or deep sleep. Surprisingly, these two states are about as different from each other as sleeping is from waking,[25] but each plays a specific role in regenerating our systems.

Why do we need to sleep?

Tomatis believes that the need for sleep is exaggerated. As the cortex needs constant energy inputs via sensory intake, and most people don't have enough stimulating activities, he thinks they turn to sleep as an escape and a refuge.

---

24 Note. This chapter was fully revised in 2009 by Rafaele Joudry, bringing it up to date with more recent scientific discoveries.

25 *Sleep mechanics,* Harvard Health Publications, October 1, 2007.

The need for sleep varies greatly between individuals as well as between species. Whilst humans need around eight hours a day, cats spend 15 hours snoozing; horses only sleep three hours, while bats hang on and doze for 20! While the hours of sleep we need for replenishment vary, there is plenty of evidence of the importance of the restorative effects of sleep.

One of the ways we have of understanding why we need to sleep so much is to look at what happens if we don't get enough sleep. It affects our personalities and our sense of humor. We may become irritable and less tolerant. Parents of small children will often say that when they're tired they get irritated at their children's antics that might amuse them if they were properly rested.

Lack of sleep clearly affects our thinking, or cognitive processes. A sleep-deprived brain is truly running on four rather than eight cylinders. If we're trying to be creative, the motor doesn't work as well. We can perform calculations, but not as quickly. We're much more likely to make errors. This is because the brain's engine hasn't been replenished.

Sleep deprivation also affects us physically. Our co-ordination suffers and we lose our agility. Sleep improves muscle tone and skin appearance. With adequate sleep athletes run better, swim better and lift more weight. We also see differences in immune responses depending on how much someone sleeps. But how does sleep achieve all this? Are there other ways to produce this type of replenishment?

Research has shown that meditation can reduce the need for sleep with no ill effects.[26] Tests done by Bruce O'Hara and colleagues at the University of Kentucky in Lexington found meditation led to superior performance in response time, even in sleep-deprived subjects. Later studies by Sara Lazar at the Massachusetts General Hospital in Boston found that meditating actually increases the thickness of areas in the cortex involved in attention and sensory

---

26 Motluk, A., 'Meditation Builds up the Brain,' *New Scientist,* 15 November 2005.

processing.[27] Similar studies have shown that accomplished musicians, athletes and linguists all have thickening in relevant areas of the cortex.

"Our data suggest that meditation practice can promote cortical plasticity in adults in areas important for cognitive and emotional processing and well-being," said Sara Lazar, leader of the study and a psychologist at Harvard Medical School. "These findings are consistent with other studies that demonstrated increased thickness of music areas in the brains of musicians, and visual and motor areas in the brains of jugglers. In other words, the structure of an adult brain can change in response to repeated practice," she explained. So it seems there is another way of achieving some of the benefits of sleep without actually sleeping. Could it be that Sound Therapy has similar effects?

Sound Therapy listeners consistently report needing less sleep, but feeling energized and well rested. Maybe the effect of cortical stimulation achieved by meditation, and in a different way by Sound Therapy, provides similar benefits to those we get from sleep. Do our sleep requirements perhaps depend on the quality of sleep we get? One question scientist have asked is, 'what type of sleep is the best?' We have two main types of sleep: quiet sleep and dreaming (REM) sleep.

Three stages of quiet sleep

Quiet sleep is divided into three stages: N1, N2 and N3. Unless something disturbs the process, in quiet sleep we gradually descend through Theta into a Delta state, known as deep sleep or slow-wave sleep.[28]

In stage N1, brain waves slow to four to seven cycles per second, a pattern called theta waves.

27 Lazar, S., 'Meditation Found to Increase Brain Size,' *Harvard University Gazette,* Jan 23, 2005, cited on 14 Sept, 2009:

http://www.harvardscience.harvard.edu/medicine-health/articles/meditation-found-increase-brain-size

28 *Sleep mechanics,* Ibid.

In stage N2, we begin to see large, slow waves intermingled with brief bursts of activity called sleep spindles. We spend about half the night in stage N2 sleep, which leaves us moderately refreshed.

Eventually, in stage N3, the Delta state, large slow brain waves become the major feature on the EEG. It is in the Delta state that your body can renew and repair itself. Breathing now becomes more regular. Blood pressure falls, the pulse rate slowing to about 20% to 30% below the normal waking rate. In this deep state it is much harder for the sleeper to be woken by external stimuli. As this stage begins, the pituitary gland releases a quantity of growth hormone which stimulates muscle repair. There is an increase, in the blood, of substances which activate the immune system, suggesting that slow-wave sleep may assist the body to protect itself from infections.

For healthy young people about 20% of their sleep time is spent in slow wave or deep sleep. However, the ratio of deep sleep reduces over our lifetime and is nearly absent for many people over 65. It is this deep, slow wave sleep which allows us to wake up feeling refreshed and is believed to be the most beneficial for restoring the body.[29]

It is very common for Sound Therapy listeners to report experiencing deeper and more refreshing sleep, while at the same time they frequently get by on less sleep with no ill effects. It seems probable, therefore, that Sound Therapy helps us to fall into deep sleep more easily and achieve a greater ratio of deep sleep during the night. One example of this was Linda Taylor Anderson, who noticed a significant difference in her quality of sleep. She wrote.

> *"When properly energized, the body can function on very little sleep. I have always required eight hours of heavy duty sleep. Now I often wake up in the night, after only three to four hours sleep, snap my eyes open, stretch and feel ready to tackle whatever may be coming my way."*

29 Ibid.

Photographer Courtney Milne said: "(Prior to Sound Therapy) I felt always harried, often exhausted and needed eight or nine hours sleep a night; now five or six suffice, and I awake deeply rested and with a supply of energy which remains constant throughout my long days." And Helen Schatzley declared, "I used to take hours to get to sleep; now, it's ten minutes!"

Dreaming (REM) sleep

The other kind of sleep, which is also essential for vibrant health, is REM, rapid eye movement or dreaming sleep. While the brain is actively creating and perceiving images, your eyes dart back and forth in rapid movement behind closed lids. During REM sleep body temperature rises, blood pressure increases and heart rate and breathing function at near daytime levels. REM sleep occurs approximately every 90 minutes, about three to five times a night. Scientists believe that REM sleep is important for restoring brain function and that it helps learning and memory.

Why is dreaming important?

You may sometimes wonder whether your dreams serve any purpose. Do they carry messages from the unconscious, symbolic learnings from the higher self, or are they simply random images thrown up by the mind at rest? Those who have studied dreaming generally fall into two camps: those who say dreams are significant, and those who say they are not.

Sigmund Freud was the originator of the psychological approach, proposing in 1900 that dreams are meaningful representations of the unconscious mind. Post-Freudian theorists focus on how dreams help the organization of thought and the consolidation of long-term memory.

Other researchers, taking a physiological approach, believe that dreams are just a series of aimless and chaotic images – little more than the mind's attempt to make meaning out of random chemical signals emitted from the brain stem.

Some recent research on the function of dreams combines the psychological and neurochemical approaches. One scientist observed that patients who had sustained injuries and lesions in the frontal lobe of the brain no longer dreamed. This suggests that dreaming must involve those areas in the front of the brain that are connected to urges and impulses, as opposed to merely occurring in the brain stem.

Many users have reported that Sound Therapy has changed their experience of dreams. Some have reported dreaming in colour for the first time, having more positive and uplifting dreams, and children have been able to leave their nightmares behind.

Dr. Cliff Bacchus, author and family doctor wrote:

"Listening to the therapy music for a time before going to sleep, I began having vivid, happy dreams, with the clarity and purity of childhood dreams: sailing away on a Caribbean cruise; flying through the high air from Hawaii to Tahiti. I also remembered the dreams in detail. At the same time, my creative doors flew open. I began rising earlier in the mornings and listening to the music during several hours of creative writing, which preceded my office hours."

Whether dreams are meaningful or not, the increase in enjoyable dream experiences seems to parallel the improved benefits of peaceful emotional states that Sound Therapy listeners often report during their waking hours.

Sound Therapy and Circadian rhythms

Circadian (meaning 'about a day') is the term used to describe people's natural sleep rhythm, which is controlled by a cluster of cells in the hypothalamus, a centre in the brain known to regulate appetite and other biological functions. Our desire for sleep is strongest between 2 and 4 a.m. and between 2 and 3 p.m.[30] Shift workers and parents have difficulty adjusting to disruptions to their sleep rhythm, as do travellers entering different time zones.

Sound Therapy appears to help us adjust more easily when these sleep rhythms are disrupted. Listeners are often surprised at how easily they adjust to a new time zone when they travel with Sound Therapy.

Don Kala, of Israel declared, "I am delighted at how well the tapes work while traveling. A journey that would leave me groggy, no longer does so. A great cure for jet lag!" And Akiki Okuwa from Japan reported, "For the first time in my life, I traveled without getting tired over the jetlag."

How the brain regulates sleep

It is possible that Sound Therapy affects the production of our neurotransmitters. The timing of our wakefulness and different stages of sleep is co-ordinated by fluctuating activity in the brain's nerve cells and their chemical messengers. Several neurotransmitters play a role in sleep regulation. Adenosine and gamma-aminobutyric acid (GABA) are believed to promote sleep. Acetylcholine regulates REM sleep, while norepinephrine, epinephrine, dopamine, and hypocretin stimulate wakefulness. People's differences in sleep habits may be linked to variations in their natural levels of neurotransmitters and in their response to these chemicals.[31] Because Sound Therapy listeners report deeper, easier and more restorative sleep, it seems probable that the neurotransmitters affecting sleep are stimulated by Sound Therapy.

Adjusting to the effect of Sound Therapy on sleep

It is the unneeded sleep which falls away with Sound Therapy. Here is what our listeners typically describe. The signal that the effect is taking hold is that suddenly one morning you wake up an hour or

30 Ibid.
31 Ibid.

so earlier than usual. You awaken simply, peacefully, feeling deeply rested and refreshed. Odd. It's six o'clock instead of seven. You roll over from habit and go back to sleep. Next time you may wake at five, then four. All the inner signals tell you you have slept enough and can get up. But you can't believe it. The habit is strong. It tries to tug you back to sleep.

The truth is you can get up as soon as you waken in that way, coming suddenly out of sleep, feeling bright and rested. You have enough energy for the day; more than enough. By late evening you still won't feel tired, even if you've been working long and hard.

Once again the habitual patterns are thrown into confusion. Do you go to bed or don't you, when you feel as though you just got up – even though it's midnight? You go to bed from a sense of duty and drift easily into sleep, without the old tossing and turning. That must mean you were worn out. Yet four or five hours later you're awake again and feeling on top of the world.

Habit tries to reassert itself, and you want to roll over and snatch more sleep, though you know very well you do not need it. An effort is needed to get up: not an effort of the body, but an effort of the will. The body is working on a new time schedule and the inner clock has to be adjusted.

Only the insomniac appreciates the full blessedness of sleep. Such a sufferer would wonder at anyone wishing to reduce that gift of gifts. But for many insomniacs, the gift is being able to sleep easily for the first time. Those listeners who reduce their sleep are only skipping the hours that it used to take to get the same benefits, for, as has been shown with other forms of music therapy and meditation, the quality of their sleep has been improved.[32] Ordinary sleep could not be cut by a third or a half. But with the energizing and tranquilizing of the system through brain recharge, sleep is concentrated and compressed, becoming more efficient. Perhaps this is the Delta

32 Cohen, L. et al., 'Psychological Adjustment and Sleep Quality in a Randomised Trial of the Effects of a Tibetan Yoga Intervention in Patients with Lymphoma,' *Cancer,* Vol. 100, No.10, 2004, pp.2253 – 2260.

sleep, deep and pure and thorough, like a child's slumber.[33]

The medical name for this kind of sleeping is hypersomnia. It is the exact opposite of in-somnia. Insomnia is caused by cortical excitation, hypersomnia by cortical inhibition – a healthy inhibition. While you are up and around the relaxing effect of the therapy manifests itself in tranquillity of mind, a sense of well-being and imperviousness to stress; when you lie down and shift your mind into the sleep gear, you sink sweetly away. The fact that you have not accumulated tiredness through the day contributes to the ease and refreshment of the sleep.

One woman, hearing how the brain recharge reduces the need for sleep, was horrified. "You want to rob me of half my sleep?" she cried. "I have enough trouble killing time as it is."

So be warned: Sound Therapy is only for people who want more time in their lives, because as sure as you listen you are going to get it. After a short period of adjustment it will become the natural thing. Then if you want to have a Sunday morning lie-in for old times' sake, go ahead. You won't be sleepy and the extra rest won't do you any good, but as the doctors say about vitamins, it won't hurt you.

Time is money, we are told. But time is something better than that. It is growth. More time means more life. There's a feeling of richness about having abundant time. It takes a pressure off the heart; no more does the correspondence pile up and the books you want to read sit nagging on the shelf. The quiet hours of darkness, when the house and street and air lanes are still, is a marvellous time for creative work, for learning a language, for studying the other things you always wanted to know. When the family comes stumbling down the stairs to breakfast, you have just hit your stride. At night when they're knocked out, you're still waiting to get tired. And you're going to have a long wait. After a while you can't remember what tiredness was. It's like the dim memory of an ancient illness.

---

33 *Lai, H; and Good, M.,* 'Music Improves Sleep Quality in Older Adults,' *Journal of Advanced Nursing,* 53(1) January 2006, pp.134-144.

The gift of extra time

At first it's disconcerting to find yourself in the living room with your cup of coffee at three or four in the morning, looking at the black windows and feeling that the sun has forgotten to come up.

You feel like asking your mother, "What am I going to do?" You know what she'd say. "Think of something."

You have to think of quite a few things. The remaining part of your life has been lengthened by approximately one sixth. If you are, say, forty, with forty more to go, you have received a gift of about six years. They can be the fullest years of all, because your mental faculties are also expanded.

For myself, the choice of reading material had always been restricted because I found so many subjects boring: a legacy from school. Especially I couldn't care about politics and history. Then one day a door quietly opened, and I became avid for politics and history. Tucking into Winston Churchill's six massive volumes on the Second World War, I found it the adventure story of the century. Next came Solzhenitsyn's horror story, *The Gulag Archipelago*. These monumental works yielded easily to the abundance of time and new receptivity of mind. Now all of history beckons. It's like opening the catacombs and scooping up the buried treasure.

I wouldn't place a bet now on what doors are permanently closed. It's not natural to have any part of the mind boarded up. And whether conscious or unconscious, opening doors never let in any spooks. Things only have the power to frighten us when they're locked out.

And look, the sun is rising.

Chapter Five

How To Listen

First, don't listen. Do something else and let the music happen without too much conscious attention – though if you want to pause and listen now and then, there's no harm in that.

You don't have to embroider doilies or under-employ your intelligence with jig-saw puzzles, though when you want to relax with such activities, it's a very good time to do the listening. In the main you just play the music while carrying on with your day. Listen at home, on the way to work – driving, walking or taking the bus – maybe even on the job, though it's likely to be more acceptable with some kinds of jobs than others. Now that the students at St. Peter's College are listening with their Sony Walkman™s five hours a day in the classrooms, the teachers are free to do the same; but don't look for it yet in the average school.

If you're self-employed, you're home free. A Saskatoon stereo repairman listens most of the day at his bench; so does a goldsmith. A chiropractor uses it while doing his adjustments and doesn't need an adjustment himself anymore at the end of the day.

To listen while reading is to impress the words more firmly on the mind, and so it's ideal for study. You can listen at meals or in coffee breaks. Try playing it at imperceptible volume while watching TV; it will give protection against that dragged-out feeling and leave you alert enough to do something useful afterwards.

For the homemaker it lightens the hours at the stove and sink, clipped to the belt or carried around in a fabric shoulder bag, or else slung about the neck. It's useful at the sewing machine or typewriter, to counteract the sound of the motor; particularly when using the vacuum cleaner or electric mixer. When the kids get too rowdy, promise them ten minutes' listening each. This should always be treated as a special privilege for children, never applied under compulsion; it's too good to ruin. It has a profound effect on the young, forming mind, and therefore is most valuable of all for pregnant women. People claim to have produced genius children by the use of Sound Therapy throughout pregnancy. Never mind genius: it's enough if the embryonic brain forms to its best advantage.

If you're a meditator you'll find it a great benefit in meditation, taking you into the deep state more easily and quickly. An excellent time to use it is after a meal, when the blood leaves the brain for the digestive system and ordinarily makes you tired; the brain recharge will eliminate the tiredness and also aid digestion due to the relaxation it gives. Play it while resting, and at night when going to sleep. If you like to read in bed, take your Walkman™ with you, and you'll soon fall asleep over your book, half waking a little later to remove the headphones and put out the light. The time that it plays during sleep is the most beneficial of all, as the sound flows unobstructedly into the unconscious mind. And you don't have to press Stop. You can set it so it goes off by itself.

Listening at low volume

Keep the volume between low and medium. It does just as much good at a faint volume as when it's louder. Since it has the effect of opening the hearing, you will find yourself reducing the volume as time goes on.

Any kind of sound at too high a level will damage the ear. We hear of young people these days destroying their hearing – what's left of it from the night clubs – by playing portable music players at top volume. This is why people will tell you that it's dangerous to drive a car with headphones on. If you can't hear the sounds around you, of course it is. But to play the Sound Therapy at low volume makes you a safer driver. It induces relaxation and keeps you alert, while still allowing you to hear the outside sounds.

And here is an important point. When you have your Walkman™ set to where you can just hear it, and you start your car or step out into the noise of the street, *do not turn the volume up*. You don't have to be able to hear the music; it is still going into your ears and doing its work. It never has to compete with other sounds.

Another reason for keeping the volume low is that you will realize all the sooner how easy it is to communicate with people and conduct all the business of your life while getting in your listening hours. At first you'll encounter resistance. People will think you're shutting them out. Simply explain that this sound is very gentle, and offer them the headphones so that they can try it.

I have found that to listen while travelling brings me to my destination without a trace of tiredness. The cause of the exhaustion that usually accompanies travel is the barrage of discharging sounds that attacks the system from the minute you enter the airport. Airports and railway stations are thick with low frequency sounds: the hum of machinery, fluorescent lights, computers, luggage carts, P.A. announcements. The plane interior emits an aggressive low frequency noise that systematically drains energy from the brain. Though the high frequency music is a faint sound in comparison, it will counteract these insidious drones, and bear us above the damage as surely as the plane itself carries us high over the earth.

Wear your Sound Therapy while shopping, unless you care what people think. If public opinion worries you, you won't be into this anyway. People may shout at you when you're wearing the headphones, but if you speak calmly back they'll get the idea.

Sound Therapy listening for children

As word gets around about the use of the Walkman™ in the classrooms at St. Peter's, the listening therapy has begun to make its way into other schools. An open and receptive attitude on the part of a few principals, teachers and parents has resulted in certain children being able to take their Walkman™ and Sound Therapy to school with them. They listen at their desks for most of the day, and reports indicate better learning, less stress, and improved behaviour both at school and at home.

And here a question arises. Some parents ask: "If I buy my child a Walkman™, how do I know that he/she is not going to use it to listen to rock music?"

The anxiety is understandable. The effect of rock music, at the volume that it is ordinarily played, is now known to damage hearing, and certainly is no aid to study. Yet the answer is simple. There are many destructive elements in this world and most of them represent one side of a coin whose other side is positive and constructive. The more beneficial a thing is, the greater its negative power is likely to be. Sound is one example; the sun is another; Creation itself has a shadow side. Wherever destructive possibility exists it exists for the purpose of being met, counteracted and overcome.

Parents universally complain about the effect of pop music on the young. But who is doing anything about it? No-one is educating young people in the effects of sound, both harmful and beneficial. Almost no-one is introducing them to the wealth of classical music that exists in the world and which will enrich their whole lives, once admitted to consciousness. To say, "Well, I'm not going to introduce my children to good sound because they might make wrong use of the music player" is to admit defeat before even trying a better way.

It is a fact that parents have been helpless before the onslaught of musical noise. Here at last is a chance to meet this threat, to educate children on matters of sound at an early age. It means granting them a measure of personal responsibility, a positive gesture in itself, and one which usually results in more good than harm.

To provide children with the means of hearing beneficial sound is not bound to encourage them in the opposite direction. At any rate, to withhold it is no protection. They are going to listen to rock music anyway, if not on their own music player, on someone else's. They're going to have their eardrums blasted at concerts or simply walking along the downtown streets. The only real protection lies in informing them and equipping them with a method of healing and safeguarding their precious hearing.

Sister Miriam at St. Peter's tells how the first students to be introduced to the Walkman™s on their desks were thrilled to death, and turned up the next day with handfuls of rock music cassettes. She saw that they had missed the point. She explained: "If you listen to Sound Therapy music for fifteen minutes and then listen to rock for the same length of time, it will undo the good effect of the Sound Therapy and take away a little something as well."

The students were interested in hearing that. No-one had ever explained such a thing to them. Most had never listened to classical music in their lives. They not only got used to it very quickly, but many grew to like it. They wanted to take the cassettes home to listen to on their home stereo systems, and a rotating library of Sound Therapy cassettes was set up. It proves again that as all the impulses of the body are toward healing, so is the direction of the mind. It only needs to be informed. To explain the differences in the values of sound, and allow young people – even very young people – a measure of choice, cannot fail to weigh the scales on the side of health.

Another question has been asked. "Are my children going to sleep less if they do this therapy? Will they start getting up at four in the morning and refuse to go to bed at night?"

The answer is No. Parents of children who are on the therapy say there is no problem with this. The listening results in a balancing and harmonizing of the person, at whatever age. Adults are relieved of stress; kids calm down. Men and women who have been sleeping longer hours than the body really requires will sleep less. Hyperactive children who have been sleeping very little begin to sleep more. Other children may have been oversleeping as an escape from emotional problems, and these will move toward normalcy with respect to behaviour and hours of sleep. Children need more sleep than adults, and therefore, when in health, will sleep an appropriate length of time. The Sound Therapy will merely assure that the sleep is fully restorative.

How many hours a day should you listen?

How long should you listen each day? There is no limit to the time that you may listen. Three hours a day is prescribed in the formal therapy, and I have found that length of time to be effective with people using my Walkman™ system. I recommend three hours *minimum,* because those who find they can manage four or five hours appear to have results sooner. Once people get into the habit of simply wearing the Walkman™ around, and it registers that they really can do everything else while listening, it's no more bother to listen five hours than five minutes. A teacher tells me, "In the morning I put on my clothes and my Walkman™ along with them. It's more trouble to take it off than leave it on. I soon forget I'm wearing it."

Note from Rafaele Joudry:

> In recent years a "Listeners Self Help Workbook" was produced to give more detailed instructions. Be sure to complete the Personalised Listening Routine Assessment, which you can look up on the contents page of the Workbook. This will give you an exact prescription for the listening routine that will best suit your needs and level of auditory fitness.

The listening does not have to be done at one stretch but can be spread out over the day and evening as convenient. It is better, in fact, to have a few breaks, to do some vocalizing – humming, singing or even talking – as the voice is also an instrument of recharge.

How much listening is required?

How long will it take? The length of time varies with each individual. The Tomatis sound therapist, by applying the listening test, can read the results on the audiogram and see the degree to which the ear's selectivity is blocked. He can then foretell with some degree of accuracy the length of time required for the opening. With self-therapy, we don't know until it happens. As a general rule, 100 to 200 hours of listening are necessary before the effect begins to be felt. A few people require less; some take longer; but if you persist there is no doubt that it will have its result.

Until the opening occurs, it's essential that you put in the hours daily. Once you've achieved the break-through, and the new energy patterns are firmly established, you can vary the listening time as you wish.

Minor passing side effects

When the ear is about to open, there's a signal. You get terribly tired. Father Lawrence has come up with a good image: "You might picture the brain at this stage as being like a bowl of jelly, held in the hands and very gently shaken." The pathways are being subtly rearranged, and as they settle into new and more harmonious patterns the new-found energy is released. The tiredness may last for a week, a little more, a little less. It's a very relaxed condition, usually coming on in the evening, and you just sleep it off. It is the last tiredness you will ever know, if you continue the regular recharging.

In most cases this tiredness precedes the inrush of vitality, but some people have been known to get the energy first and the tiredness later – or not at all. There is a period, on the cusp of change, when you should refrain from playing the music while driving, for you could drop off to sleep. There could also at some point be a slight aching of the ears; this is due to adjustment of the middle ear muscles. It's a sign that the Electronic Ear is changing the nature of the auditory system and is a good sign. It will soon pass. Some people report a touch of dizziness from time to time, and this passes too.

The great difference in the speed with which people respond is due to a number of factors, such as the extent to which selectivity is blocked, and also whether the person is an audio or visual type. Some people relate to the world through their ears, and others through their eyes, and there are extremes and variants of these. A purely audio type is likely to experience the opening of the ear much faster than the visual person. Musicians are already halfway there, in contrast to visual artists, whose ears can be very stubborn.

Right-brain/left-brain responses

Visual people tend to be "right brained" – more strongly influenced by the right hemisphere, where the spatial sense is located. As the right hemisphere is influenced by the left ear, such people are more comfortable with a predominance of sound to the left rather than the right. They are sometimes very resistant to the Sound Therapy music with its right ear emphasis, and when nobody's looking might switch the headphones around!

The left hemisphere, in the overwhelming majority of people, (mirror image twins are an exception) contains the centres for language, memory, concentration, and the active force for the release of energy. The hemispheres are equal in importance, but their activities are different. The right hemisphere may be visualized as the instrument, with the left taking the role of virtuoso, or the one which executes. The right hemisphere is marked by a force which is receptive, while the left is invested with consciousness and activity and becomes the dynamic representative of the central nervous system.

Writers, and people dealing in language and symbolic thought, appear to respond more quickly than others to the opening of the auditory system through this therapy. Yet it may be that those whose ear is slower to open are in need of it most. Their selectivity may be blocked on all frequencies. Little by little the uncultivated areas have to be cleared and brought to life. Though it takes longer, the end result will be all the more gratifying and worthwhile.

Technical aptitudes are a function of the right hemisphere, and in my own case, I can only consider that for most of my life my right brain was pretty well out of commission. I was hopeless at drawing, couldn't do math, had no spatial sense, tending to misjudge distances and bump into things as I made my way around. The radical effect of the therapy on my grasp of things technical indicates clearly how the sound, though directed to the left hemisphere, affects the brain in its entirety. It would also seem to conform to Tomatis' statement that, due to the differing lengths of the circuits, stimulation directed to the left hemisphere reaches the right by a shorter route than if fed to the right, via the left ear.

Therefore we are encouraged to tend the right ear to all sounds. In conversation, try to seat yourself so that the other person's voice comes from your right. I leave it to you to imagine the fun when two sound therapists start jockeying for position!

Sound Therapy recording methods

About the Sound Therapy albums: All are recorded with right ear dominance, so it's important to put the headphone marked R to the right ear. After a time this emphasis begins to sound natural, and your normal music, with equal balance, will seem rather strange.

Each of the albums is filtered to ascending frequency, starting at normal, rising to anywhere from 3,000 to 8,000 Hz, levelling out for a while and then returning to normal. This aids the ear in tuning itself gradually to the high frequency sound. Once adjusted, it can accommodate a steady 8,000 Hz, and some more advanced albums maintain that frequency all the way through.

Variety is an essential factor in our lives. Listening to this for three hours a day makes it essential to have a wide choice of music. The program should never be attempted with a single album: after listening to it daily for a week, you'd never want to hear it again. Sound Therapy is available as a series of programs each consisting of several albums. The programs are used progressively to create a gradual and cumulative opening of the ear and re-charging of the brain.

Though the filtering varies on the albums, they are recorded from first to last through the Electronic Ear, and it is this device which distinguishes Sound Therapy from several other high frequency systems, or simple Music Therapies. It is the 'rocking effect' of the Electronic Ear which exercises the middle ear and opens the auditory system to the full range of frequencies. Somewhat similar is the Bates method of strengthening the muscles of the eyes through exercise. Very few people are willing to stick with those exercises, because they're boring. They're something you have to do, whereas the Electronic Ear does this for you. Its unique sound is detectable on the album as a faint, intermittent hissing, rather like snow striking a window. It may detract from the purity of the sound, but is doing a world of good, and so the sound has to sacrifice a little.

Equipment for Sound Therapy

When Sound Therapy was first released, portable playback on analogue tapes was available and was the best portable music delivery system for the therapy. Many changes in music technology meant that in 2006 a version was developed on CD, being careful to retain the full frequency range and integrity of the analogue original as much as possible. However, MP3 (often referred to as I-pod™), though portable and convenient, does not, at the time of this printing, have a good enough playback quality for Sound Therapy. New high quality digital solutions will develop in the future and Sound Therapy International will always make the therapy available on the best high quality uncompressed playback system available. Check with your Sound Therapy consultant for the current system.

Sound Therapy recordings are made on analogue equipment which preserves the high frequencies and tonal qualities of the music.

Never compromise the quality by attempting to download or make copies of your program, but always play it in the original form as provided.

High quality headphones are important so that the full range of high frequencies will reach your ears. Follow the current recommendations of Sound Therapy International to get the best results.

The listening must be done with headphones, though it is possible to play the music through speakers and derive a slight benefit. It might be tried in a room where children are playing. As children are particularly responsive, they may get almost as much from it as an adult with closed hearing listening through phones.

If two people in the house are doing the therapy, they shouldn't try to share a music player – or even a battery charger. The main feature of the self-therapy is the freedom to listen when you choose, and relationships could come to grief through wrestling over the equipment!

Long-term listening

The time comes when the effect is more or less permanent; the auditory system has been changed and acts, as it were, like a dynamo recharging the central battery, which in turn distributes energy to the whole nervous system. You will have learned to tune into the high frequencies wherever they exist. Linda Anderson, the writer, says: "I'm charged by everything now – my regular music, my own voice, the voices of others, bird songs and the sound of rain."

Beneficial long-term effects

Once you are experiencing the Tomatis effect, you can then suit yourself as to how much listening you want to do. Extra demands on your energy can be met by putting on the high frequency music. While there is a consistently higher energy state, there's no reason to suppose that that level cannot be steadily lifted by continued use of the music. Some people become so fond of the sound that they choose to go on listening to it every day, and look forward to doing it for the rest of their lives. The effect appears to be cumulative. As the energy level maintains its high state and imperceptibly rises, the relaxation deepens into a yogic serenity, an imperviousness to stress.

Beneficial 'cat naps'

Once the auditory opening has occurred, there is a little technique for using your new long days to fullest effect. When you feel yourself slowing down, sit (or lie) back with a book and your Sound Therapy and read to the music. Your eyes will grow heavy; very soon they will close and you'll sink down into a mini-sleep which may only be two or three minutes but will be as refreshing as an hour. You will awaken fully alert, with none of the hungover, groggy feeling that usually follows a daytime sleep. Doing this occasionally, you will find that you never have to come to a long full stop – that is, unless you want to.

But at the start there are two rules that can't be emphasized too much.

First rule: Regular listening is essential

The listening must be done regularly. "Spot listening," picking it up now and then, is useless. To do it halfway will not give half results: it will give no results at all. Compare it with a weight lifter lifting weights. The muscles must have the daily, unremitting exercise if they are to develop. It is the same with the development of the middle ear muscles, those which bring about the transformation in listening and cause all the rest to happen.

Second rule: Change happens gradually

Don't look for quick results. Allow two to four months before expecting to notice any change. The occasional person takes much longer. It is a process, a re-education of the ear, not Aladdin's lamp. Some people put on the headphones for five minutes and say, "It isn't doing anything for me." That's like picking up a foreign language textbook and flipping through it with your thumb and saying, "I can't speak the language yet." The new language of frequencies has to be acquired, and the rates of speed are as individual as individuals themselves. Some listen for a month or two and then fall into discouragement because someone else made the breakthrough in half the time. The other person was probably predominantly left-brained, an audio type, and lacked the childhood traumas that contribute so much to closing off the receptivity of the ear. The longer it takes for the ear to open to the recharging effect of the high frequencies, the more the life force has been dammed up and the more essential it is to release it. Only the very exceptional person starts responding within a few weeks. Everyone wants to be exceptional, so will hope to fall into that category. If you're doing Sound Therapy at all, you are exceptional enough.

The initial effect can be dramatic, but don't count on it. More often than not it's a gradual thing. The new energy comes creeping in; the expanding glow is subtle. You're feeling terrific – but can you be sure of what's causing it? Skeptical people invariably cast about for every reason under the sun that might explain the unaccustomed vitality and serenity. It's the moon, or some new medication, or maybe self-hypnosis – until the day comes when they can no longer deny that it is the Sound Therapy and nothing but the Sound Therapy. Once openly acknowledged, enthusiasm grows and before they know it they're trying to convert all their friends.

The Recharging effect of the voice

The Hindu mantra, "OM," is based on scientific knowledge of voice vibration and its energizing effect upon the brain, particularly the pineal gland for awakening intuition. The real value is in the end "mmmmm" of the "OM," which sets everything vibrating, with the mouth closed and the tongue blocked inside the mouth.

The Tomatis therapy incorporates this principle in a humming technique which is introduced after the selectivity of the ear begins to open. The microphone and headphones are used, so that the voice comes back into the singer's ears, with greater volume to the right ear. Try it after a few weeks of home listening, and you'll find it will add to the effect. You hum – any tune within the mid-range of your voice, and you can test and find the best range by paying attention to the degree of vibration it sets up in your head; notes too high or too low will not cause as much vibration. The mouth should be kept closed and the lips projected forward poutingly; this eliminates tenseness at the corners of the mouth, as tenseness of these muscles inhibits the functioning of the middle ear muscles. This forward thrusting lifts the humming vibration up into the head, and you can test this too, by humming with the mouth open or the lips held normally; you will feel the difference. You can then add to the effectiveness by lightly holding the right ear closed, or even putting a little cotton into it; thus you get the right ear emphasis.

If you feel foolish – and who wouldn't? – do it while alone in the house or on solitary walks. It's good for gardening, and for walking on the beach, where you don't want to take your Walkman™. And it's a lifesaver when you run out of batteries.

It would seem from this that deaf people would be very deficient in energy. It is true that they have to work harder than most of us for their supply of life force, and some are able to rise to the extra demands which are placed upon the brain, and others are not. There is a certain compensation in that the deaf are not prey to the low, discharging sounds which bombard the hearing person. But there is work to be done in exposing the hearing-impaired to high frequency pulses and also in training their voices for the recharge that accompanies humming.

A silent order of Monks

To illustrate the importance of voice vibration, they tell the story of a silent order of monks in France. Forbidden to speak, they had always sung for six hours a day. But even monasteries have a young generation which is protesting against the old ways, and at one point the monks decided to abolish singing. They couldn't see that it had any particular purpose and was a waste of time, six hours a day and eight on Sunday. They did away with song, and right away they got tired. Investigating the cause of their exhaustion, they decided it must be their habit of early rising. They took to sleeping in in the mornings and got even more tired. They revised their diet, thinking that possibly they should start eating meat like everybody else. Their energy levels sank lower, and some months after this experiment began, Dr. Tomatis was called in.

He arrived at an abbey that contained ninety monks and found seventy of them sitting in their cells doing nothing, withdrawn like schizoid beings. He knew immediately what the problem was. With his electronic equipment he began re-educating the monks' ears and restoring the ability to sing. That was in July. By November, sixty-seven monks had begun to be active again. For the other three nothing could be done; they were advanced in the disintegration of their being and ended up in a mental hospital. Their brains had become completely discharged through lack of stimulus, and could not be sparked back to life. It makes you think. It makes you sing.

So now, knowing all the rules, you are ready to begin. But don't, we repeat don't, expect the results to be strictly by the rules. Any good therapy takes account of the differences in people, and Sound Therapy more than most allows for tremendous variations in the type and speed of response. This has nothing to do with brains, or spiritual evolution either. It is simply the marvellous, mysterious uniqueness of people.

You will not necessarily experience the 'breakthrough' we speak of, but maybe only a 'creepthrough'. You may only have improved sleep (only!) or better hearing, or reduced stress. It's a gamble. But whether you win a big prize or a small one, you will win something. You can't lose if you just put on the headphones and walk, man.

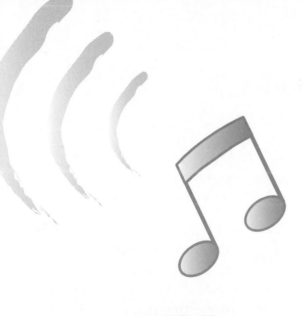

PART II

Listeners Stories

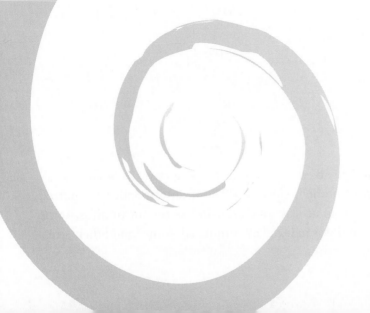

Listeners' Stories

> 66 *Listen, my son, to the voice of your God, and open wide* 99
> *the ears of your heart.*
>
> The first Rule of the Order of St. Benoit

Some people ask, "Have you done scientific tests with Sound Therapy?" Twenty-five years after the portable method was first released we are in a position to report on the experience of many thousands of successful listeners. Three surveys have been completed on the home-based listening program between 1991 and 2009 and each indicated that 80 to 90% of listeners benefited in a variety of ways.

The results from the initial survey were as follows.

Condition	Percentage that reported Improvement	Sample size
Tinnitus	86%	187
Hearing loss	56%	123
Energy	84%	122
Stress	86%	80
Sleep	75%	127
Communication	78%	71
Dizziness	70%	30
Speech problems	64%	14

Most respondents benefited in one or more ways, so looking at all the benefits combined, close to 90% of all respondents reported a positive result in at least one area. In the case of tinnitus, some found the sound was reduced or eliminated, some found their stress levels and their reactions to the tinnitus were reduced. Eighty-six percent of those with tinnitus found the therapy helped them in some way.

Although it was not a controlled study, this mail survey, where listeners responded voluntarily, does give a good indication of the type of results people may experience. It also clearly indicates that responses to the self-help program are very similar to the results achieved in the Tomatis clinics. To see a full research summary on studies done on the Tomatis method and various other research papers you can visit www.SoundTherapyInternational.com/Research

More scientific research is needed in many areas to explore the effects of the therapy in greater depth, and with increasing interest in Tomatis's work worldwide, we hope to see this happening in the near future.

Some of the responses people have are dramatic, some subtle. The following pages give many examples of the letters we have received over the years, and continue to receive. Certain effects turn up in almost all reports: the improved sleep; the relaxation, energy and sense of well-being; also, frequently, the improvement in listening or more focused hearing. Sound Therapy may be of great benefit to the blind, due to its sharpening of the hearing faculty, and the possible protection it gives against hearing loss with ageing.

And then, other people have something uniquely theirs to add – asthmatic attacks allayed, and in a couple of cases a sense of taste returning after being completely lost for years.

Some reported a change in eating habits saying that the increase in energy motivated them to exercise, resulting in greater fitness and even weight loss. In a few cases chronic pain was alleviated and energy increased, so exercise happened spontaneously.

Our understanding of this diverse range of benefits is now supported by new research on the brain. In recent decades, a fascinating new field of scientific enquiry has uncovered the mechanism that

111

allows all these changes to occur. The new field of brain plasticity has prompted numerous laboratory experiments proving that our sensory experiences, our reactions and our aptitudes can all change when we stimulate the brain with the right sort of sensory input. More on this in Part Three. But the clear fact emerging from this new field is that everyone has the capacity to change their brain. This means that with persistent and consistent use of Sound Therapy, everyone who has ears to listen will reap the positive benefits of this therapy in their own unique way.

The reports are not all in, and will never be all in as long as there are unique individuals out there walking around with their headphones on. But here are a few samples chosen from many. All of these individuals have gladly given their permission for us to print their stories.

North American Stories

Linda Taylor Anderson, author of Carousing in the Kitchen, Melbourne, Florida, U.S.A.:

"My friend Patricia didn't endeavour to convince me to give Sound Therapy a try. It was my own idea. I wanted what she had: extra energy, more waking hours and blessed tranquillity. That is why, as a healthy, functioning person, I incorporated Sound Therapy into my life.

After less than sixty hours of listening, suddenly, incredibly, new sounds were singing in my ears. I had assumed I'd always heard them, but it is amazing how much we hear, yet do not hear. I am now acutely conscious of sound, all sound, including my own voice which I can now control. Octavizing up or down is now easily accomplished. It is Sound Therapy that has gifted me with this new awareness. Further amazement came. When properly energized, the body can function on very little sleep. I have always required eight hours of heavy duty sleep. Now I often wake up in the night, after only three to four hours sleep, snap my eyes open, stretch and feel ready to tackle whatever may be coming my way. I do not always rise to the occasion, preferring the comfort and warmth of the bed. But there is none of the old tossing and turning. I lie peacefully, pursuing my ranging thoughts, making promises and programs for the hours and days to come, as I am now able to concentrate my energy into a basic force that is not easily sidetracked. I see others fade; I am fresh and eager for the next encounter. If I feel the approach of tiredness, I simply lie down for a few minutes with the music and drift into rest, rising calmed, refreshed and ready to carry on."

A year later Linda writes: "I'm still listening. Not three hours a day but at least 45 minutes. I usually listen at night; when I go to bed, on go the headphones. I go to sleep and the music plays on. When I miss a day I'm not happy about it. I feel something important is lacking. It's as though my internal batteries that provide calm, energy and a feeling of well-being just hadn't been charged. I'll never stop listening. Never is a strong word, but that's how I feel about Sound Therapy. I never want to be without it."

Darrell Johnson, Delisle, Sask., Canada:

"About four years ago I started getting ringing in the left ear, followed by light-headedness and dizziness. Sometimes I couldn't stand without falling. This I was getting about once a month, then twice a month, soon twice a week; and not long later three or four times a day. My doctor told me I had Meniere's Syndrome, which is a problem of the inner ear past the stirrup. There wasn't much that could be done; I would just have to put up with it. As my age was 53, I knew I would be quite some time putting up with this problem. The doctor made some changes in my diet, which helped a little but not much. It was no cure, and I still got the spells. Then I heard about Sound Therapy. I bought the Sony Walkman™ and Sound Therapy albums on June 15th. I played it three to five hours a day. It took about ten weeks before I noticed any difference. Now, four months later, I have no light-headedness and dizziness, and

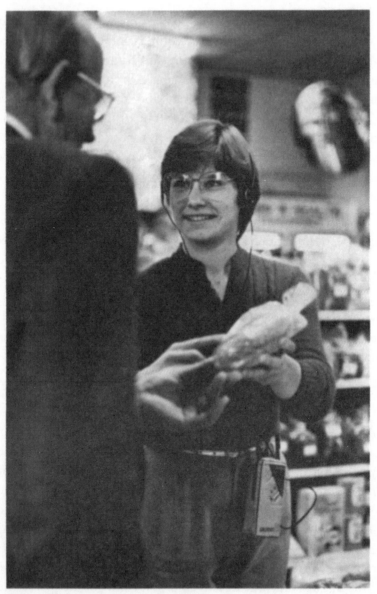

Donna Hagel listening while serving in her health food store and tuning customers into the therapy, Saskatoon, 1984

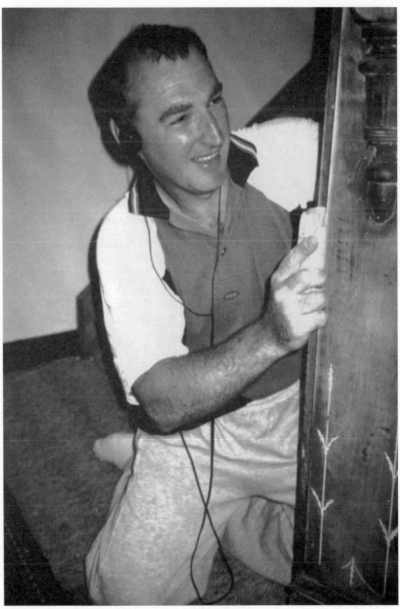

You can listen while working around the house

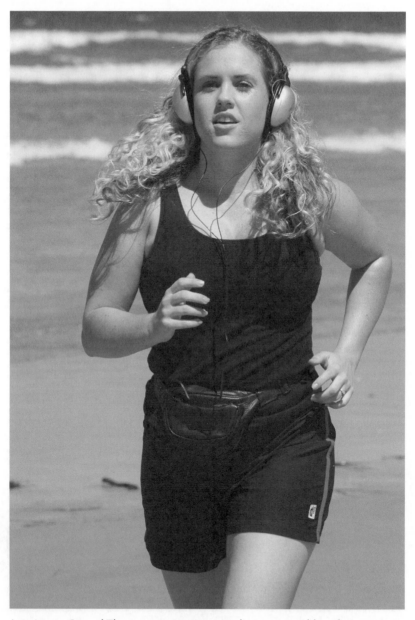

Jogging to Sound Therapy means greater distances and less fatigue

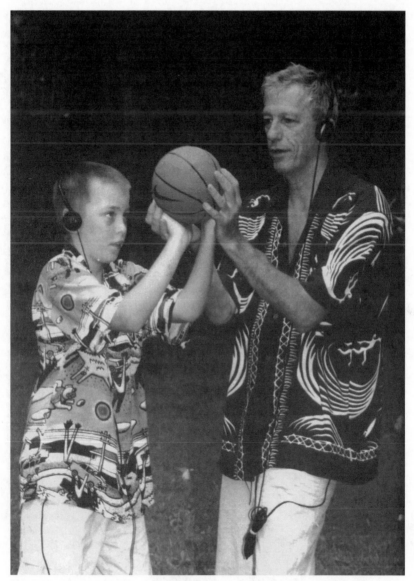

Listening during play improves communication and co-ordination

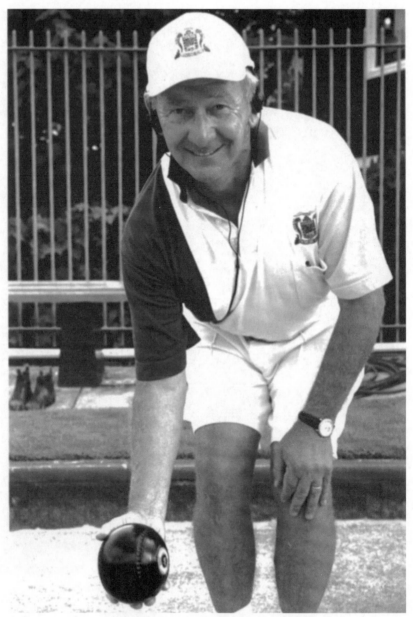

Balance and spatial distance are enhanced by using Sound Therapy

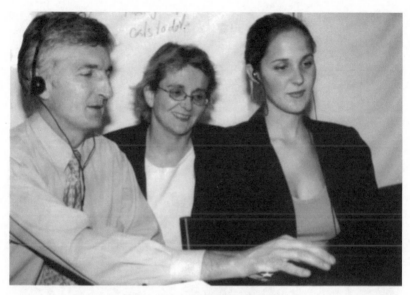

Listening at the office keeps the mind focussed and alert

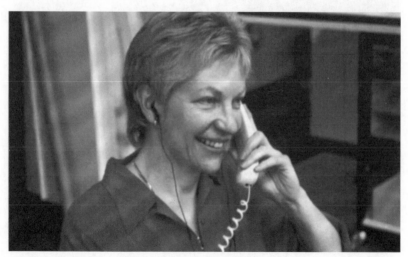

Listeners find they end the day feeling energised instead of exhausted

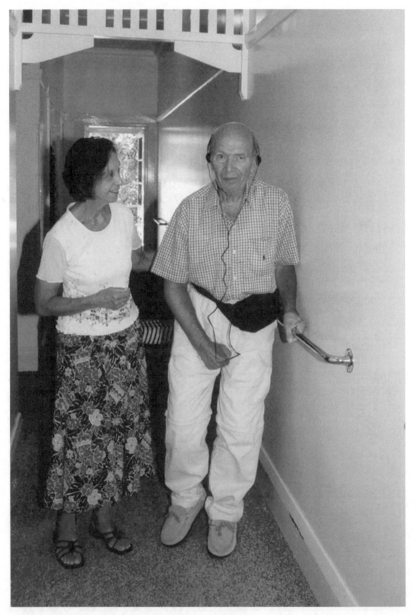

Sound Therapy stimulates the brain to help patients regain mobility and speech after a stroke

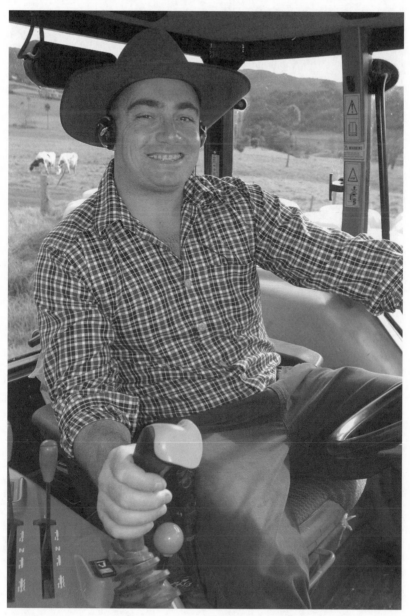

Farmers reduce fatigue and stimulate the brain by listening while driving the tractor

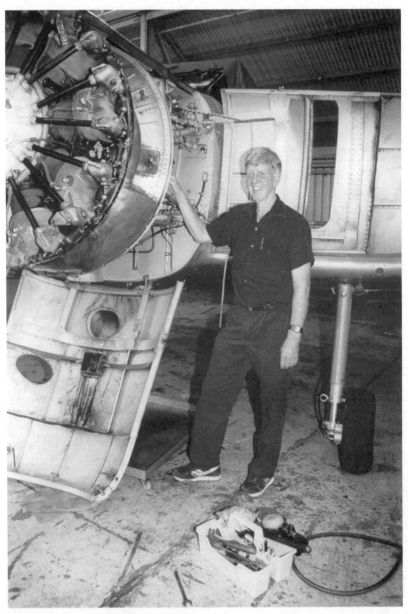

Pilots need to look after their ears which may be damaged by aeroplane noise and changing altitude

the ringing in my left ear has gone. Sometimes I get the feeling that I might get dizzy, and I put on the Sound Therapy music and the feeling goes away immediately. The hearing in my left ear has also improved. I can't express how much Sound Therapy has done for me. I still listen three to four hours a day, as it is so relaxing, and I am never dragged out and tired any more. I can stay up very late at night and still get up rested early in the morning. Also, I don't get uptight and stressed about the little setbacks of the day, but can just relax and take them in my stride. I even find it easier to talk to people – am not so shy! It's like a new life."

Courtney Milne, photographer, Saskatoon:

"Since the Sound Therapy has taken effect for me, I no longer know what anxiety is. As a photographer, lecturer and writer, I am travelling continually and am bombarded with more than average demands. Even at the times of greatest pressure I feel an inner calm, a peace and tranquillity that lifts me above the stresses of the moment. I have no doubt at all that this is due to the therapy, as I compare my present state with that of a year ago before I began the listening program. At that time I felt always harried, often exhausted and needed eight or nine hours sleep a night; now five or six suffice, and I awake deeply rested and with a supply of energy which remains constant throughout my long days.

Although I experienced the opening of the ear some months ago, I still listen for several hours daily, as I enjoy the music and it keeps my energy unflagging, my peace intact. I find it extremely simple to wear my Walkman™ almost anywhere without it interfering. I drive, jog, read, listen to the radio, carry on day-to-day conversations, eat my meals and do my photography while listening to the music. I would not be without it when writing as it is conducive to creative thought, the music humming along unobtrusively like a built-in mantra.

Sound Therapy also puts attention on caring for myself. It has had an influence on my eating and drinking habits and my desire for regular exercise – a strengthening of the positive life wish. For example, as a moderate social drinker, it struck me one day that I have no need of alcohol to relax me or make me happy – so why drink any? I now jiggle my ice in a glass of fruit juice and no questions are asked except the usual one: 'Where do you get all that energy?'"

Students at St. Peter's College, Muenster, Canada:

Here are some brief comments from students at St. Peter's College, after a few months of listening to the portable Sound Therapy program issued by the school:

Susan Stroeder: "I enjoyed this therapy and learned to pay more attention in school. I wake up easier in the morning – my Mum doesn't have to call me anymore. I don't have to ask questions twice, but hear things the first time."

Kyle Bauer: "I don't get headaches now and am much more active."

Marian Niekamp: "Don't need as much sleep and am not tired in the mornings. My speaking is much clearer."

Keith Carroll: "It made me much more calm and relaxed."

Lyle Witt: "My right ear seems to bug me when I listen to hard rock now."

Debbie Nagy: "I've been listening to Sound Therapy for over 600 hours. I find it very relaxing. I can sleep a lot better at nights. I wake up more easily in the mornings and find myself in better moods. I don't mind listening to it at school, and on weekends I try to get as many hours as I can. I find I can study a lot better and I'm more prepared for tests. I'm really enjoying the classical music."

Norman Altrogge, University student and part-time restaurant worker:

"Over and above assisting me in relaxing and winding down, my hearing became much keener as I listened to the music from day to day. There followed improved concentration and it seemed easier to zero in on things. The listening had a sort of snowballing effect in improving my ability to focus my mind and put myself into whatever I'm doing with a larger degree of intensity."

Claude Heppell, Rimouski, Quebec, Canada:

"The most recent effect of my Sound Therapy, after 14 months of listening, is rather amusing: for I have lately discovered an ability to do crosswords, at which I had slaved in vain in the past.

As a purely visual person, it took me a long time to realize effects with this program. I was patient and persistent, as I enjoyed the music and found that I missed it when I skipped a day. Gradually I found myself becoming a more social person, feeling more and more love for others, with a powerful new capacity to interact and create in volunteer groups for old people. I am 46, and whereas one might say this was a natural maturation, I believe that, on the contrary, change is more difficult as we get older.

A few months ago, singing some folksongs for my own pleasure, I realized I had more ability to strike the right notes than before. And when I speak, my voice, which I disliked until recently, is gradually becoming more resonant, warm, and well controlled. All thanks to the Sound Therapy listening program."

Mrs. Helen Schatzley of Thompson, Manitoba, Canada:

"I used to take hours to get to sleep; now, ten minutes.

I do my husband's bookkeeping, often having to work whole days at it. Those days used to be very stressful – I had all sorts of upsets and made many mistakes. I now wear the headphones the entire time I'm working on the books and get through it like a breeze, with no mistakes.

The main effect of the Sound Therapy has been on my blood pressure. For years I had high blood pressure, 160/100 being an average level. After about two months listening to the Sound Therapy with a Sony Walkman™, my pressure began going down. One day during my checkup the nurse read my pressure and said, 'Wait a minute, I'll have to get another machine, this one isn't working. There's no way your blood pressure is going to be 120/80.' But that's what it was.

Some months after that I went through a terrible time, caring for a demanding invalid, who called upon me day and night. I didn't put on the headphones during those weeks as I was afraid I might miss hearing her. (Now I know that crisis times are exactly when I should keep up the listening.) My blood pressure shot up to 225/127. After it was over I started listening to the music again and my pressure came down 50 points in the first hour! It soon returned to normal.

My doctor was amazed. 'What have you been doing?' he asked. I showed him the book. He has now taken me off medication.

Not only that, but my hearing has improved tremendously. When I started the listening, I had to have the volume on my Walkman™ set at five or six – now I listen at a setting of one-half.

My husband is now doing the therapy and for starters has stopped snoring!"

Mrs. Schatzley sent a photograph of Dr Schatzley and herself with their Walkman™s and headphones – and a third family member, also wearing phones. She explains that their little cocker spaniel was hyperactive, and as the therapy has been so useful with hyperactive children, they decided to try the headphones on their dog. She says: "To our astonishment, the dog will sit and listen endlessly, remaining perfectly still. If we put any other music on her, she lifts her paw and knocks the headphones off."

Others might find it merely amusing, and some traditionalists might scorn this use of the therapy; but a dog is endowed with inordinately sensitive hearing and suffers from harmful sounds as much, or more than humans. This little cocker spaniel could be opening a door to a vast area of comfort and healing for animals of all kinds. They don't all have to wear headphones! Considering an animal's sensitivity, the music might be played softly over speakers in places where dogs are penned up in kennels, relieving their desperation and misery. Animal lovers can take it from there.

But it takes a dumb creature to know a beneficent sound when it hears one.

Carla Gaunt:

Carla is a brain-damaged, mentally handicapped teenager in Saskatoon, who has been doing Sound Therapy for the past three months and loves listening to the music. Her parents report that there has been a great improvement in her ability to handle stress; her speech has developed and also her recall of past events.

Maureen Boyko, Watson, Saskatchewan, Canada:

"Our son, Mitch, is going to St. Peter's Pre-Vocational Centre in Muenster. He has been listening to Sound Therapy on a Walkman™ in school since he started there last September and we've had the program at home since our purchase in April, two months ago.

Sister Miriam, one of Mitch's teachers and also principal of the school, said she has noticed a real change in Mitch in the final two months of the school year. My husband and I have noticed a real difference as well. His posture has improved. He used to walk really slouched. We're not reminding him to stand straight nearly as often. He is more relaxed; he speaks out more clearly and more often. He used to speak so softly and did not articulate his words clearly. He feels that he has much better sleep, listening to the music. And last but not least he has developed a real appreciation of classical music."

Herbert Spanier, Toronto, Canada:

"My immersion into the world of Sound Therapy has had several positive results. A strikingly noticeable one was in my work as musical performer and composer, where my creative potential was dramatically opened up. The compliments I am receiving for my concerts, where improvisation is a key, are more numerous and enthusiastic, and this from contemporaries and audiences alike. Also in the areas of stress and fatigue, considerable modification is being observed."

127

Dan Stuckel, Red Deer, Alberta, Canada:

"Before I began using the Sound Therapy my hearing was becoming progressively worse. Ear specialists told me it was caused by nerve damage, therefore nothing could be done for me. They said the ringing in my ears would become louder as time went on, thereby reducing my ability to hear. I purchased an 'in the ear model' hearing aid after I found their predictions to be correct. My hearing did indeed deteriorate. I found I had to wear the hearing aid more and more as time went on, to a point where I was wearing it 80% of the time.

After about three weeks of beginning the Sound Therapy, the ringing in my ears began to subside. Along with that my hearing also began to improve. One day I felt something almost like a minor earthquake taking place deep within my ears. Since then my hearing has improved to such an extent that I seldom have to use my hearing aid. I am able to function quite well without it now, after seven months of Sound Therapy.

To list a few of the other benefits from this therapy: I am able to sleep better and can do with much less sleep than previously required. I am doing less needless worrying, and stressing situations are much easier to cope with than they were before. In fact my entire well-being is showing a vast improvement."

James W. Bragg, Kentucky, U.S.A.:

"Sound Therapy has transformed my life. I've been listening to the program for two months, and while I started feeling subtle effects almost immediately, the real change occurred about five weeks into the program.

To give a brief history: I have spent a lifetime surrounded by a good deal of noise, but always had sufficient energy until about 1972. I was building my house and using power saws and an assortment of very loud motorized tools. After less than a year of this, my energy level dropped to virtually nil – five minutes of work followed by thirty minutes of rest. It got progressively worse, and

I was very worried. Loud sounds drove me frantic.

I teach piano at Morehead State University. Piano playing became extremely difficult for me. It got so I could hardly stand to do it. I have played publicly only three or four times since then, with three to five-year rests between performances, and I was *never* satisfied with the results. It always seemed as if a short circuit existed in my expressive mechanism. I was aware of a lack of connection in the heart area and the parallel area in the spine, and worked very hard to *think* it together. Needless to say, it never worked.

Well, let me tell you! My sound has changed, and I *love* to play! The playing experience has been transformed. I seem to be hearing back the sound that I go for, and that affects the way I make the next sound. The musical cycle is now complete. With the experience of musical sounds being so greatly deepened and expanded, I am liking music which previously bored me and adoring music which I previously liked OK. The implications for the learning and teaching of music with this therapy are vast.

Then, for many years I have had great trouble with my shoulders, upper spine and neck. It was never comfortable and the shoulders often painful in the extreme. Yoga made it worse. Activity hurt. I was a virtual cripple. I began to see a chiropractor, who said my upper spine was severely misaligned. During this period I began the Sound Therapy. At between five and eight weeks he was mystified to notice that the natural curvature of my spine was fully restored and assured me that he had not done it. He said he had never seen or heard of such a thing and would probably be drummed out of the profession if he wrote it up for a medical journal. My posture is transformed and I have real shoulders at last! This is obviously reflected in my playing since the shoulders are extremely important in piano playing.

In addition, I have had an elusive speech problem since childhood. Sometimes the speech was fluent and easy; other times it simply would not come out. I literally could not talk. Most people were not aware of it, since I 'cleverly' disguised my problem by acting 'professorial' – thinking a lot and talking very little and slowly. All of this had a devastating effect on my personality, creating mood swings which were violent and unexpected. As a result, depression became an old, old friend.

Now this is all changed. *I can talk!* Mood swings are very mild and no longer a problem. I truly feel that I am being myself for the first time in my life. I know who I am. Energy is greatly increased; stamina and endurance greatly improved. I sleep from two to four hours a night and awake feeling marvellous.

Just call me Lazarus!"

Wanda S. Harrison, Allen Park, MI, U.S.A.:

"I did experience the energy breakthrough. For about a week prior, I had found myself literally at loose ends, unable to make decisions, not really wanting to do ANYTHING. On Tuesday the 17th, I had to force myself to get up at 10:30 a.m. and dragged through the rest of the day and evening. The next morning I awoke feeling like a new person, so full of energy I couldn't decide what to do first. This is a new experience for me! I simply can't believe how much energy I have! When we were up at my mother's old farmhouse in Midland last weekend, I not only cleaned inside the house, but got to work in the yard, pruning the bushes that hadn't been done for 10 years and finally getting started on the huge task of cleaning up her old garden at the side of the house.

For the first time in many years I am able to lie down and go to sleep without taking any pills! This alone makes me feel like a new person, not to be tied to the bottle of tranquilizers at bed time; and particularly to wake up after four to five hours of sleep feeling totally refreshed, and no morning 'blahs.'

I also find that I no longer need to use laxatives the way I did for many years since I had abdominal surgery when I was seven. My memory is much clearer, as are my thought processes, as well as my writing ability."

Donalda Alder, Teacher of the Hearing Impaired, Long Beach, CA, U.S.A.:

"The children's poetry album, *Let's Recite*, has been a Godsend for my hearing impaired students. They love it! Their attention spans have increased dramatically since they have been listening regularly to the program. My one very hyperactive youngster has settled down to her schoolwork because she knows she can listen to the album as soon as she's finished. Sound Therapy has become a reward!

It's amazing to me that for the 35 years that I have been teaching hearing impaired children, this is the first auditory training program that uses only speech to which the children can listen comfortably. Patricia's speech is articulate and soothing. You have chosen the poems carefully so that they are amusing and hold the children's interest as well."

Cynthia Connell Davis, West Warwick, Rhode Island, U.S.A.:

"Specifically, I can testify that within a week after beginning my listening to the first album I was able to write the plot for a novel. I have never before been able to envisage a plot for fiction, though I have been able to write all other aspects of fiction. (Don't try to imagine my frustration.)

Apparently I suffer from a mild, erratic but progressive dyslexia and a reversal of (brain) sphere dominance.

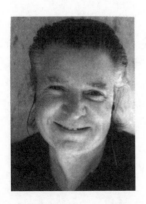

Improvement – as well as more patience, better listening capacity, more empathy for my writing students, decreased anxiety and depression and fatigue has been steady. I am tremendously enthusiastic about Sound Therapy."

Kevin Pleming
had tinnitus for 35 years. After six weeks of Sound Therapy it stopped completely and has not returned, eight years later.

131

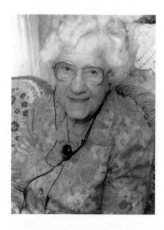

Gladys Irwin
began using Sound Therapy when she was 87. Not only did it help her hear better but it gave her new energy so she said, "Even walking up hills is easier!"

The Australian Experience

Melanie King, singer-composer, Melbourne:

"I have had some beautiful benefits from using Sound Therapy – trebled energy, less sleep needed, steadier moods, more focused concentration – and I have notes in the top of my vocal range which are brand new."

P.S. Some months later: "My voice continues to soar eaglebound in new ways!"

Allen McNeil, New South Wales:

"I am amazed at the power of this method. After just six hours I noticed benefit in my energies, and played better tennis."

Flick Evans, Somers, Victoria:

"I began to suffer from tinnitus and had received medical advice that nothing could be done about it. I read the Sound Therapy book from cover to cover at least four times, and each time put it down – convinced that it was just too good to be true.

I mentioned it to a member of our local library, who told me that her daughter was using the program and "…wished that she had started two years earlier." So I decided to try it, without any great hopes or expectations.

I had been listening for approximately 100 hours when I suddenly became aware that the tinnitus whistle had stopped – I wasn't sure WHEN it stopped – but it had. Since then I have periodically been aware of the whistle but by relaxing my head muscles for about two minutes – it disappears.

About the same time I noticed a distinct improvement in hearing in my left ear – there had been noticeable loss in that ear for about three years.

I had a client who served in the Royal Navy during the last War – in gun turrets on board ships in action. His hearing was affected to the extent that one had to raise one's voice when conversing with him. After my hearing improvement I started talking to him about Sound Therapy – and eventually found him with his own Walkman™ and music albums. A few weeks later I received a phone call at 11:00 p.m. one evening. It was my client – and his message was: "I thought I would ring and let you know that I have just heard my wife's Microwave 'BEEP' for the first time." 'nuff said!

I do not know what response others will get from the program. I can only say that I have been VERY, VERY satisfied."

Andrea Blackman, Kiama, New South Wales:

"Four years ago I developed a problem with blocked Eustachian tubes whenever I flew. Not being able to hear people properly was very frustrating, irritating and isolating. Any pleasure in attending events was replaced with anxiety at not being able to be myself as I had to struggle so much with being attentive to conversations. Occasionally, this problem would rectify itself on the return flight as the plane was taking off but eventually I would suffer for weeks (then months) at a time with blocked ears. This problem persisted until I decided to use Sound Therapy a year ago.

When my ears "popped" within three days of starting the treatment, I realised that my hearing had been worse than I thought! I cannot express the relief of having my hearing restored. Irritability and that strange sensation of disorientation simply evaporated with it. An unexpected benefit occurred in the second week of treatment – very tight muscles in my jaw seemed to uncoil, leaving me more relaxed. I have also noticed that I no longer clench my teeth during the night. How wonderful!!

I have flown many times since starting Sound Therapy and have not had painful ears or blocked Eustachian tubes. Besides, I also ensure that this will not recur as I listen to Sound Therapy when I fly, so enjoy the other benefit of arriving refreshed and energetic. Sound Therapy is such a wonderful experience in so many ways."

William A. Whiteside, Toowomba, Queensland:

"My hearing was progressively deteriorating and my social life disintegrating as I could not possibly concentrate on a conversation in an environment with a cross-current of various conversations. When trying to sing in church I could not hear my own voice, and so gave up trying. Whereas I used to enjoy music, now it just existed and gave me very little lift. I had to try so hard to distinguish any words a soloist was singing.

Road noise drove me frantic. The noises I did not want to hear became a maddening roar, and those I wanted to hear I could not.

After listening to Sound Therapy all this is changing. It brings tears of gratitude to my eyes, this recharging of life, made possible by this wonderful therapy. I can now hear the timbre in my own voice as I sing equally with that of others, and I can even hear the birds singing as I walk in the park. I am using my hearing aids less and less.

It is more than just improved hearing though. I find myself able and willing to communicate with people, it is easier to smile and reciprocate love.

During my life I have experienced a series of great personal traumas. These have left me with a tendency towards depression, sometimes quite severe. Some of these traumas were the result of my own errors, and some were caused by events beyond my control. Every time something occurred to bring these memories back I became depressed. I know that the past needs to be faced and dealt with, and with the opening up of the mind that this therapy helps to achieve, I am finding that the beauty of music enables me to know that God loves me, and first and foremost wants for me His peace. This means that when memories are recollected I can experience healing without the strain of self-effort, and a whole new experience of restored life is the result.

The deep significance of the scriptural emphasis on music, specially in the psalms, becomes very obvious.

I hope these words are an encouragement to the many thousands of people suffering from this same complaint. I never want to be without my precious Walkman™ and the therapy program. For me it is the best invention since the wheel."

Ruth M. Arnott, Beechworth, Victoria:

"I am quite sure that the program has been beneficial in releasing tension and enabling me to sleep better and therefore to think and work better. I no longer suffer from a periodic depression of feeling weighed down; especially it is helpful when I have finished teaching my piano students, the tension and fatigue are released somehow.

I am very happy to report that within the last month I discovered that I am not deaf on arriving at Wodonga/Albury or Wangaratta, which are considerably lower than Beechworth! It was a real thrill I can assure you, and when coming back to Beechworth I did not feel the pressures in my head when climbing back up the hill.

I used the therapy on my return plane trip to Auckland and was thrilled to find that at each destination I had *no hearing problems whatever!* It was incredible in view of my lack of hearing on previous journeys, and I can't say enough in praise of my all round benefits when people ask me what I am doing! It has given me courage to attempt further travels. My family too are continuing to reap benefits."

K. Joseph Biggs, Burleigh Heads, Queensland:

"Looking back over past years, I have come to the conclusion that somewhere in my childhood, I closed off my hearing level to a point where the darkness of retreating eventually overcame my ability to want to hear.

By the time I was 35, I had passed through some of the most disastrous years of my young life. About that time I contracted an industrial disorder where industrial noises repeat in the hearing long after the noise is out of range. Within the next four years, I made an appointment (out of sheer frustration) with a specialist who performed a stapedectomy (An operation to replace the stirrup bone in the middle ear with a prosthesis.)

I say categorically, no person should be subjected to this dangerous treatment before being alerted to the alternative treatment which Sound Therapy provides.

I was always mentally drained, the numbness was still there and there seemed something pressing on the ears which affected my ability to hear. My doctor shrugged his shoulders and said the audio test was the same as that taken about four years ago.

I commenced Sound Therapy in January 1991. After about 200 hours of listening every day I noticed some changes, headaches diminished, tiredness fading, less restless sleep. Shoulder and back pain reduced, posture improved, better sense of direction of sound, improved sense of balance. Hearing improved, fuzzy noises in ears not so apparent.

Previously, trying to talk to a group of people in a room was nearly impossible, and a one-on-one conversation always brought signs of rejection, when everyone else thought that they were not part of the conversation.

I have now clocked up 444 continuous days for a total of 2043 hours, and now average about three-and-a-half hours per day. You don't have to be sick to gain the benefit. One very noticeable benefit is the correlation between resonance in the voice and the ear. If you can hear better, you can speak better.

Noises in the ear, (by the way aggravated by an operation) at times now reduce to zero. I am not embarrassed by noisy locations, or entering into casual conversation. Sometimes there is pain in the ears, but this soon passes. There is a reduced need for sleep, about six hours per night is sufficient, whatever may have been necessary previously.

I'm able to express thought better, do not tire easily – have more energy, posture improved, mental alertness, self-confidence, better concentration, more relaxed – but alert, some dizziness – it soon passes.

There is no doubt in my mind, the findings of Dr. Tomatis are widespread, with outside noise levels discharging our energy; and childhood problems being carried into adult life. A great deal of credit must go to Patricia Joudry for her effort in making the treatment available."

Hans Wuelfert, Lavington, NSW:

"When I was in the German army in January 1944, I had an infection of both inner ears and the Eustachian tubes. Because my temperature was only slightly elevated I was given a few Aspros. The greater part of the problem became chronic.

A year later I was a gunner in a light armoured car. During gunnery exercise there was a malfunction in the 2cm. gun which caused some kind of explosion. Fortunately all the hatches were open, but I had little hearing or sense of balance for a few days.

The result of both incidents was tinnitus with a combination of sounds; a waterfall, ringing and static. My eardrums tended to feel sucked in, quite uncomfortable at times, often I could not pop them out when I blew my nose with nostrils blocked.

In 1979 a sinus condition developed which I blamed on the type of chalk I was using as a teacher. My singing tended to be out of tune.

The range of notes became narrower. For many years I suffered from tiredness which I now attribute to some degree to the "low-frequency noise."

In January 1987 I had encephalitis and myelitis endemic to the Murray Valley. At one stage the resulting symptoms were called the M.E. syndrome: chronic lack of energy; diminished long-term and short-term memory, self-inflicted stress, pronounced sensitivity to variations in atmospheric conditions.

After two months of Sound Therapy (330 hours) this is my assessment:

Sinus condition has improved gradually and is about 80% better in general.

Eustachian tubes improved about 50%

Left ear, much lighter noise of a higher pitch, almost pleasant compared with the original noise. Congestion far less, about 70% better.

Right ear; very slight ringing, higher pitch, some congestion left, about 90% better.

Hearing in general has improved. All the sounds are crisper. At the dentist the "new" crisp sound of the drill nearly made me happy.

Singing: during walks along the open road, there is a "resonance space" again in my head, singing is in tune again and I can correct a wrong note.

Deep refreshing sleep. Requirements shortened by 1-2 hours.

Energy seems to have increased, I find it easier to start something, have a bit more go.

Memory has improved slightly. Words of some forgotten songs have come back and dialing a phone number is a lot easier.

Generally speaking, I feel that a considerable change has been going on within me and apparently still is."

John Long, West Pennant Hills, NSW:

"Many years ago my wife and I were members of the local UC church choir until we had a choirmaster whose voice I just found impossible to hear. The choirmaster who succeeded this one was worse in that I could not comprehend his Scottish accent. We both left – I because I could not hear properly; and my wife also as she was not able to drive the car, through failing eyesight. She is 84 and I am 86.

We are regular church attendees and I used to love to sing the good old hymns, but this was not possible because as I know – the larynx only accommodates what the ear hears.

Well, having read the Sound Therapy book again I decided to give the therapy a go and after about six weeks I was surprised one Sunday morning to discover that I could sing again. I have also discovered that I could once again whistle and hum aloud and recognize what I was humming."

Julia Angel Gulenc, Moorabbin Victoria:

"About eight years ago, I read an article in a women's magazine about the damaging effects of loud noise on our hearing. Sound Therapy was mentioned. Since I was suffering from frequent ringing in my ears, was very sensitive to noise, with frequent headaches etc., I rang the phone number given on the article.

I read the book in one sitting. I was so impressed, that immediately after reading it, I purchased the program. I have said many times since, that the few hundred dollars I spent buying the Sound Therapy kit was the best investment I ever made for my health. From the very first moment I started listening, I knew it was going to be good for me.

I had for a very long time been very uncomfortable listening to regular music with headphones on, as I found it unpleasant no matter how low the sound, it bothered me. Not so with Sound

Therapy. As soon as I put the headphones on, after only a few minutes, I knew I was onto something different.

I couldn't get enough. I listened for six hours straight. That same night I slept with my headphones on. I was amazed and very pleased.

A few months later, the ringing in my ears, my regular dizzy spells, and my headaches, were largely gone. I felt so energized that I went from needing eight to nine hours sleep a night, to only seven. Many times since, I have woken up feeling fully rested after only or six hours of sleep.

Now years later I don't listen every day and I don't need to, but if I go without them for longer than a fortnight, my ears seem to protest and on come the headphones again. I enjoy the music – especially the hissing; would you believe? – that special sound will continue to be a very important part of my life.

Sound Therapy has certainly made a great difference to the enjoyment of my life. My ears and I are very grateful."

Julie Wentworth, Malvern, Victoria:

"I am writing to tell you how pleased and surprised I was with using my Sound Therapy on a flight from Melbourne to Rome in April, 1996. This was my fourth flight to Rome and I could not believe how fresh, alert, and energetic I felt as I walked off the plane, and into the terminal.

When tired, I find in forty minutes, I am "recharged" and refreshed with listening to my Sound Therapy.

I believe in miracles, and am conscientiously writing down my hours each day, to keep the record of the day; and of the 300-hour mark, and the 600-hour mark.

The use of Sound Therapy all the way to Rome, and on the return flight gave me a tremendous energy boost at my destination. I will never travel without my Sound Therapy."

Mrs A Stolz, Kirwan, Queensland:

"A note to let you know how excited I am at the results I have with Sound Therapy. After approximately 20 hours of listening, I believe I am experiencing positive results.

I am a Registered Nurse working in a neonatal unit where we care for sick and premature babies. There is a lot to learn and know in this relatively new field of nursing. Because each baby's weeks of gestation, present age, and weight must be considered before starting anything else, I felt my mind was in a fog for a long time in working out their progress. Now I find a joy in being at work that I haven't had before. It is a marvellous feeling.

I have been listening to my Sound Therapy very softly, just before I go to sleep, or sometimes, on days off, while doing housework. I play it softly so I can listen to the same album many times without tiring of it before I change to another one. I look forward to 100 hours of listening and have put on layby Walkman™s for all the members of my family including grandchildren.

Thank you so very much for making this therapy available."

Nevell Phelps, Moree, NSW:

"I suffered from tinnitus for several years until it reached the stage where it was difficult to go to sleep. I consulted a doctor who advised that there was nothing that could be done to cure the problem. My wife then bought me a set of four of your Sound Therapy albums. After several months the annoyance had abated considerably and for years now I haven't had the slightest sign of it returning.

Thanking you for your incalculable assistance in the past."

Patricia Jankovic, Kirribilli, NSW:

"At a very difficult time in my life, I was introduced to *Sound Therapy*.

It certainly improved hearing loss in my right ear and reduced tinnitus.

My sense of well-being improved greatly. I was not aware of how unhappy and stressed I was until I started to experience a feeling of happiness inside and a more balanced emotional state.

Being a shift-worker in a health profession I have noticed better quality of sleep and I am able to be more focused. I truly look forward to long walks with my Sound Therapy. Somehow I am able to appreciate more the beauty around me.

Sound Therapy will continue to be an important and special part of my life."

Sarkis Doueihi, Sydney, NSW:

"My name is Sarkis Doueihi, I am a personal trainer and full time Athlete (competing in Track and American Football). I studied psychology at California State College Fullerton, and NLP at Master practitioner level with Wyatt Woodsmall & Marvin Oka.

My greatest passion is performance enhancement, to see human beings becoming and being the absolute best that they can be, whether that be in sports, business, family, relationships, or even the spiritual path.

I first came across Sound Therapy while reading *Cosmic Memory* by Sheila Ostrander and Lynn Schroeder. The chapter on using the ear to recharge and learn just knocked me out. Firstly, because of its claims, secondly, because of evidence and background, but most importantly, to the extent that it described certain things I had experienced. I must have read and re-read the chapter at least three times, then exploded to the back of the book, looking for the resource listings, only to find an address in far off Canada. I didn't want to wait weeks and weeks to get the Sound Therapy program. I wanted it now or at least by the next morning. I was sure there had to be an Australian connection.

Funnily enough the next day a catalogue arrived in the mail for the upcoming Mind Body & Spirit festival (Dec. '94). As I flicked through, my jaw dropped, there right in front of me was a local phone number for a supplier of Sound Therapy, and they even had a stall at the show.

On the Thursday of the show I rushed straight to the Sound Therapy stall. The cosmic joke was that here I met the daughter (Rafaele) of the originator of Sound Therapy for the Walkman™ (Patricia Joudry) and she lives in Sydney. On that day I picked up the book *Sound Therapy for the Walk Man*. I read it from cover to cover in one sitting. Now was I hyped. I wanted this therapy and all the benefits that come with it.

In the first week I must have listened to in excess of 70 hours, I was so excited I literally lived with my Walkman™. It took me about four weeks to hit 300 hours of listening and when it hit me the fatigue was phenomenal. Sitting in front of the TV after a pretty ordinary day, it was only 7.30pm and off I dozed. For the next two weeks it was pretty much the same. I would wake up exhausted, I would fall asleep at the smallest rest break or inactivity. It wasn't like I couldn't continue with my daily schedule of training or working, it just took a lot more effort and concentration on my part. I was tired all the time and when I slept, I slept like a rock. Then my ears started to ache, all the dizziness and deep bone soreness! Despite all the fatigue and aches, all the dizziness and confusion, I persisted. I knew there was a pot of gold at the end of this colourless rainbow and I persisted. As suddenly as all the symptoms came, they one by one disappeared, but as each disappeared there was a gift of some new ability.

The fatigue, for example, was not only alleviated, it was totally gone, with energy to burn. There was this new intensity to my workouts, my work had a new spark, and my life felt energised. When the ear-aches dispersed there came a new sense of balance and proprioception (awareness of the position and movements of the body). There was clarity in my brain, not just in my mind. I had so much energy and more than anything I became totally addicted to my Sound Therapy. I seemed to feed on it.

About two or three months later I ordered the advanced program. I listened to it for about 100 hours before it all started to happen again, but from a higher order, the symptoms came on for only five days this time, and the after-effect escalated the original by at least four fold. I was so energised, so earful it was great! Like my hearing seemed to get deeper and wider.

And I noticed more than ever how I slept like a baby, totally stress free. Most of all I seemed to be able to feed off all the sound around, not only the Sound Therapy. I was always energised.

What next you ask? Well I tried the Full Spectrum audios and was totally blown away. They have a depth, a dimensionality to them like nothing I have ever heard. To describe them in words almost seems impossible, because to hear them is to go beyond the horizontal mind, into a verticality beyond words.

Sound Therapy is performance-enhancing, it is life-enhancing. If you are after truly getting an edge on yourself then it would pay you handsomely to try the Sound Therapy experience. Persist through till the end and you will be swearing by it too."

Letters from Around the World

Dr. Cliff Bacchus, author and Member of the American Academy of Family Physicians, Governor's Harbour, Eleuthera, Bahamas:

"I was introduced to the Sound Therapy portable system and began listening to the music on the day that I purchased my Sony Walkman™ in Miami. I listened for about six hours a day during the first three days, while making my way about through the noise and confusion of that city, and also during the flight back to my island of Eleuthera. After these three days I was aware of an energy and mental clarity such as I had not experienced since before entering University, many years earlier. One notable happening during the first week was that, whereas I had never before had the patience – or stamina at the end of a day of seeing patients – to play backgammon with my young daughter, as she constantly pleaded for me to do, I could now spend a whole evening with her at this game, wearing my headphones and listening to the therapy music. Thus, there was an immediate improvement in family harmony. After ten days of listening, there was a change in the character of my dreams. I had had great difficulty in remembering my dreams, while knowing that they usually verged on the nightmarish. Listening to the therapy music for a time before going to sleep, I began having vivid, happy dreams, with the clarity and purity of childhood dreams: sailing away on a Caribbean cruise; flying through the high air from Hawaii to Tahiti. I also remembered the dreams in detail. At the same time, my creative doors flew open. I began rising earlier in the mornings and listening to the music during several hours of creative writing, which preceded my office hours. I now sleep better, think better, write better, and am eager to get all my patients onto Sound Therapy – particularly the pregnant women, and the children with learning problems."

Don Kala, Israel:

"I am delighted at how well Sound Therapy works while travelling. A journey that would leave me groggy, no longer does so. A great cure for jet lag!"

Patricia Proenza, Finchley, London, U.K.:

"There have been changes, which I hardly dare believe are happening. There has been a reawakening of the musical 'spark' within me. Having been trained as a pianist and taken a degree in Music and also composed, my life seemed to fall apart in my early twenties, when suffering a severely strained shoulder which didn't seem to get better. This was accompanied by mental misery and there seemed to be a gradual withdrawing of the creative energy, as playing was always accompanied by physical pain and mental anguish. As life got more complicated in many areas I gave up piano teaching and stopped practicing, since there was no spark there, no desire. Only pain and guilt at not having developed a God-given gift.

That was fifteen years ago, so what is happening now, the beginning of a reawakening, is for me a miracle. Although physically much stiffer and with aches and pains, I am so thrilled that the fire inside has been re-ignited, even if it is a small flame. I have recently composed a piece of music, which although not in original style, is at least a beginning.

I have realized too that I have improved mentally – I seem to be more positive, brighter, and much less prone to feelings of despair, unworthiness etc. My friends have noticed quite a difference in me – more than I have, as the changes have been gradual."

Annaliese Palsans, Ahrensburg, Germany:

"It's a wonder! Your Sound Therapy has helped really. One morning, it was the 22nd of August, I suddenly noticed that the noises in my left ear had gone. I switched on the television to look if the speakers' words are more clear, and they were. I couldn't believe and knocked on wooden things – Germans do that to make sure that a situation will stay long. I didn't tell Jurgen but the whole day I put the buttons in and off the ears to make sure there are still no noises. Up to this day I have no noises in the left ear and can hear very well the whole day. At first my doctor wasn't very interested. But the audiogram tells him the truth. My left ear is as good as it has been before all the trouble began. He has never had a patient whose ears had become better again, when they had been as bad as mine.

Two weeks later

I'm still happy, for the good success goes on. Now the right ear, too, starts to get better. There are still noises but I can hear the music on a lower condition so by and by there changes something too.

Friends of mine often tell me that I'm now again this person they have known before I became ill, though I thought I had never shown how desperate I was. They must have noticed it."

Cecily Bova, Cape Town, South Africa:

"At last I am able to send you my experience of Sound Therapy. I have been listening for up to six hours a day since October last year (five months). A truly hard case with very stubborn ears. I am not just a visual type, but an artist, deciphering everything through my eyes. Without being told, I already knew I was 'locked in,' for that is how I have experienced the world, as though I lived at a distance: which makes sense because the eyes are the furthest-away sense.

I loved music, but I knew the quality of sound evaded me, and I longed to hear as a musician would. Much as I enjoyed colour tones, rhythms, I knew my ears were not experiencing true sound.

Being a dyslexic adult, with switched off ears, has caused terrible suffering, as you will understand. I am in my mid 50's and it has taken all these years to wait, and work only with body and eyes, cut off from true sound.

I have experienced a lot of anger and frustration, because of the loneliness and isolation: one of my main hang-ups in the world was that I felt invisible. In fact I was beginning to call myself the invisible man (woman). I was ignored, in other words. My anger was in my voice. No doubt all who heard me would switch off.

The results came and went. I kept a diary for three months. Everything stressed me in the end, change of life, the terrible South African situation with the increased isolationism of that, stressful home situations, homesickness for England, and hostility for South Africa made me feel more locked in than Mandela.

Last week a change began to take place. I could not sleep a whole night. I was wide awake... my mind clear and active all night. I was frightened by it. Then awake all day, with no fatigue. This has continued, my mind clear, not disturbed. My ears are lighting up. In the past two days I am aware of them as appendages on each side of my head, my ears feel like horns, or shells, I feel their depth into my head. Sound is coming through, I am "switching On", Patricia, with a calming effect. I can hear the anger in my voice. My speech has become softer; I am so amazed by this listening ability. I keep on thinking it will stop. If it does I'll go mad.

At last I am aware of the other, the thou in my life. There is no doubt about it. Sound Therapy in my case acted like First Aid. I was drowning, like a stranded whale, disoriented, I missed that quality of being bathed in sound. Supermarkets, noisy places, and loud pop music drove me insane. I lived purely with my eyes, focusing on colours and enjoying life in the artistic manner. Any disturbance of that made me angry, critical and aggressive. I always felt as though my privacy was being invaded.

Now my experience of Sound Therapy has humbled me. I am in awe of sound. I can actively focus on sound sources. It's incredible, as though I have been given a new instrument, calming my mind and soul.

Bless you, Patricia, and all the brothers who helped you and worked with you to produce this for the man in the street. I could not have afforded the therapy in a listening lab."

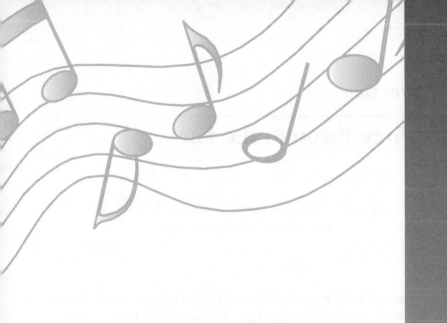

PART III

The Latest Developments

By Rafaele Joudry

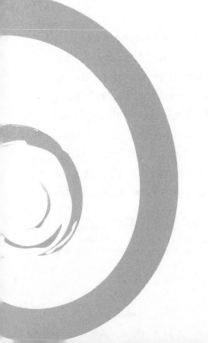

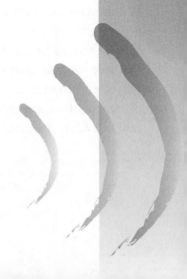

Chapter One

Journey through the Ear

> 66 *This machine trains athletes of the middle ear –* 99
> *it produces champion listeners.*
>
> Tomatis

This chapter is for people who would like the physiological facts about the ear and brain. We have treated rather light-heartedly a very serious and complex subject. This is partly because light-heartedness is the essence of the effect itself, and also because to treat it with the seriousness and complexity it warrants would make it inaccessible for a person not trained in the sciences of the ear.

The important thing about this technique is to do it; that's all that matters. It is not necessary to grasp all the complexities of Audio-Psycho-Phonology in order for the method to work for you, but this chapter aims to make the process more knowable for those who wish to know.

The explanation put forward in this chapter is based on theories proposed by Dr. Tomatis to explain how Sound Therapy works. While many of these ideas are not yet proven or accepted in the general scientific arena, those who have examined them closely have found them to have merit. A thesis by Dr Weeks in 1989 explored the role of the complex interconnections between the cranial nerves and the ear and how this may account for the great range of benefits listeners report from Sound Therapy.[1] Dr Richards in 2004 developed a neurological theory to explain how responses by

---

1   Weeks, Bradford S., 'The Therapeutic Effect of High Frequency Audition and its Role in Sacred Music,' *About the Tomatis Method*, eds. Gilmor, Timothy M. Ph.D; Madaule, Paul, L.Ps; Thompson, Billie, Ph.D., The Listening Centre Press, Toronto, 1989. See Appendix 2.

the middle ear muscles come under the control of centres related to auditory function in the brain. [2]

Health professionals who would like a more detailed explanation are also directed to the Appendix by Dr. Weeks M.D.

Which comes first, thought or language?

Our brain evolved over millions of years, paralleling the unique accomplishment and aptitudes of human beings. Tomatis has posed the idea that the evolution of our language abilities is what gave us our humanness: that in fact our capacity for human thought springs from our language skills. This is somewhat of a chicken and egg question. Does thought create language or does language create thought?

Tomatis would go as far as to say that language builds the brain.[3] The development of our brain begins long before birth, though our complex web of neural connections continues to develop throughout childhood and the rest of life.[4] The miracle of our brain is its ongoing state of plasticity and resilience. Thus our education and enculturation serves to continue our evolution into independent and self-aware social beings. It is through the vehicle of language, the means of most sophisticated human communication, that this development continues to shape the brain.

Even before birth, the speech areas of the brain are highly developed. The left hemisphere of the brain, the area of the cortex dedicated to speech, is larger and more developed in 65 percent of human brains before birth. The speech function is firmly located in the left brain in 95 percent of the population before the age of five.

So we can see that we have a biological predisposition for language.

---

2   Richards, G; Richards, P.J; & Joudry, R., 'The Therapeutic Effects of High Band Pass Classical Music and Antioxidant Supplements,' Presented to the Australian Audiological Society Conference Brisbane, 2004. Cited on www.SoundTherapyInternational.com/research

3   Tomatis, A.A., *The Conscious Ear*, Station Hill Press, New York, 1991.

4   Tomatis, A. A., *The Ear and Language*, Moulin, Ontario, 1996.

The physiological organ systems that we use for language are specific to the human species. They enable us to convey and conduct sophisticated cultural learning and interpersonal communication.

Our brain delivers, interprets and makes sense of our perceptions so that we can recognise colours, shapes and sounds and recognize sensations such as hunger, pleasure and pain. Our amazing web of neuronal connections in the cortex (the conscious brain) miraculously turns electrochemical impulses into conscious perception.[5] And as we receive these perceptions they are simultaneously charged with emotional feeling in response to our subjective experience. This instant humanizing of our awareness means that all our perceptions are subjective and personalized by our interpretation of incoming stimuli. Perception depends on our interpretation and so, by definition, it cannot be "objective."

When we say the brain is "plastic" we mean that it is constantly malleable and changing. Its very structure forms as a result of sensory input.[6] Through our own thought or mind training, using techniques such as yoga or self-hypnosis, we can learn to inhibit sensory inputs and thus reduce our emotional reactivity. It is even possible to eliminate pain with such techniques. On the other hand we can increase our acute perception of certain pleasurable stimulation, by turning down or blocking our awareness of competing stimuli.

Tomatis has shown that a child, being much more attuned to bodily needs, may choose to close down to certain outside stimuli which seem unpleasant or daunting. The danger of such tendencies is that the child also unwittingly shuts out stimuli that are needed for its development. It is well known that in children deprived of human interaction and nurturing we often see a severe lack of emotional and cognitive development.

The explanation given in the following pages is drawn from the works of Dr. Tomatis and his two colleagues Dr. Bradford Weeks

---

5   Greenfield, Susan, *The Human Brain*, Phoenix, London, 1997.
6   Doige, N., *The Brain that Changes Itself*, Scribe Publications, Carlton North, Vic, 2008.

and Dr. Agatha Sidlauskas who have written elegant explanations elaborating on Dr. Tomatis's theories.

Organization of the ear

What surprises people most about Sound Therapy is that so much can be achieved, simply by listening to sound. Surprise gives way to wonder as soon as one understands the miracle of the ear and the integral role it plays in our entire functioning. The inter-relatedness of ear and brain is the key to understanding the remarkable range of effects of Sound Therapy. We know that all matter vibrates. The vibrations of sound that we can consciously hear, are simply those of a particular frequency – or speed – that resonates with the ear.

Dr. Tomatis has made us aware that the ear is not simply a collector of outside information. It is an intrinsic and essential part of the development and active functioning of the brain and the nervous system. As one of the primary sense organs, the ear is orchestrated and controlled by the ingenious Central Nervous System. The ear is part of, and is an organ of, the Central Nervous System. As such, it has a remarkable degree of involvement with the cranial nerves: those nerves which issue directly from the skull through separate openings. In fact the ear has been called "the Rome of the body" for almost all of the twelve pairs of cranial nerves – numbers 2 to 11 – have some traffic with the ear. [7]

Following a sound vibration into the ear

To take a journey into the inner chambers of the ear, let us follow the course of a sound vibration as it navigates the complexities of the hearing organ. Imagine that you are a sound vibration on your way, via the ear, to the brain of the listener. The listener could be seen as a large and complex organization, and you, the sound vibration, are a messenger seeking a meeting with the director.

First you arrive at the outer grounds of the organization. This is the skin and the outer ear, the part you see on the side of the head, called

---

7   Weeks, Bradford S., Ibid. See Appendix 2.

the pinna. Even as you enter the driveway – the outer ear canal – the organization is alerted to your presence. The surveillance system picks you up and relays the warning to watchers in the organization that a sound is coming, for the outer ear canal acts as the security system to prevent unwanted sounds from gaining access to the inner chambers. This occurs not through means of a door, but through an early warning system.

Further in we will meet two doors, and both have been alerted now to the incoming sound. The wiring of the ear's surveillance system consists of two of the cranial nerves. The 5th and 8th pairs of cranial nerves communicate with the outer ear flap (the pinna) and so the brain can alert all the muscles intrinsic to the ear that a sound is coming. Will it be a welcome or an unwelcome guest?

Well, that is a question for the receptionist. The receptionist, of course, sits at the front door, known as the tympanus or ear drum. (The ear drum, is a flexible membrane much like the vibrating skin on a drum, which separates the outer ear canal from the middle ear.) Will she or will she not permit entry, and how will she decide?

The receptionist (ear drum) is linked up to an extraordinary network of information so she by no means has to judge the visitor on face value. First there is the vagus nerve, (the 10th cranial pair, named vagus for the vagabond or wanderer.) The vagus is a communication channel to many parts of the organization (or organism).

The branch (or twig) of the vagus nerve which lies across the ear drum would appear incidental, except that it means the ear is party to the many other ports of call that the vagus makes. In the throat the vagus communicates with the 9th cranial nerve, the glossopharyngeal nerve, sharing responsibility for the speech mechanism, (movement of the tongue and throat.) The receptionist is thus linked in to the intercom system. Next the vagus contacts the spino accessory (or 11th cranial nerve) transferring its messages to the spinal column and the postural muscles. The receptionist thus has knowledge of the outward appearance and public image of the organization.

The Ear

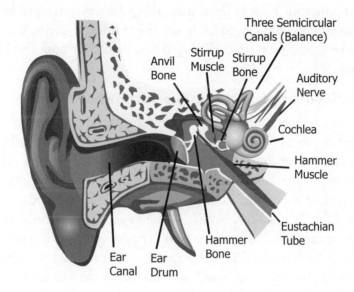

The vagus then proceeds on down to innervate the bronchi and the heart (supply them with nerves,) so the very breath and vital needs of the system are within earshot of that good woman at the reception desk – the ear drum! Finally, after joining the opposing vagal nerve, the vagus plunges through the diaphragm and connects to the entire viscera – the lining of the intestinal tract from oesophagus to anus. It also communicates with three of the sacral nerves at the very base of the spine. This means that there is very little going on (breath, digestion, posture, heart beat) in terms of the organism's needs of which the receptionist of the ear is not informed. Her decision as to whether to admit the sound, as you can see, is not made without due consultation.

There is more to the story, for she is also instructed from above by the Director (the brain), but more on this later.

Suppose the visitor is deemed unwelcome, what happens then? Behind the receptionist (the ear drum) is an air-filled chamber known as the middle ear. The only opening is the Eustachian tube leading into the back of the throat. This tube serves to equalize the pressure between the outside air and the middle ear cavity. You can experience the pressure balancing if you hold your nose and blow gently.

Tomatis's description of how sound is processed in the ear

Here is one theory of what happens when sound reaches the ear, according to Dr Tomatis and his advocates.[8] In the middle ear chamber is a chain of three tiny bones called the ossicles. These bones serve as a link between the ear drum and the inner ear. The first two of these, the hammer and anvil, serve as guards to the front door. The hammer muscle – *tensor tympani* – controls the ear drum in degrees of tenseness as well as positioning. If the incoming sound is too intense, defences are set up. The ear drum (tympanus) tenses up. The inner ear, which we could see as the Executive Team, is alerted. The Executives send a message back to the guards (the hammer and anvil) to close the gate, and the ear drum is relaxed so the incoming sound vibrations are blocked. At the same time the mouth opens, equalizing the pressure in the middle ear cavity in correspondence with the outside stimulation on the ear drum, and: "I am sorry," the receptionist says sweetly, "the Director will not see you today."

If, on the other hand a decision is made to admit the visitor, the hammer muscle (muscle of the guards) is used accordingly. The ear drum – receptionist – then adjusts her demeanour and ushers the visiting vibrations to enter the mastoid bone, for bone conducts sound as efficiently as does air.

The mastoid is one of the solid bones that form the skull. The ear drum is mounted around its circumference, directly on the mastoid bone, so if the ear drum is correctly tuned, the vibrations pass easily into the bone.

8   Tomatis, *The Conscious Ear*, Ibid.

Here our story, which is drawn from Dr. Tomatis' theories, adds some new elements to standard, orthodox theory. Orthodox theory portrays the hammer and anvil as conveyors of the message, conducting the sound vibration to the third little bone, the stirrup, and from there to the inner ear. But in Dr. Tomatis' view the hammer and anvil clearly play a guardian role and act as advisors to the receptionist, but not conveyors of the sound.[9]

The stirrup

The third of the little bones in the middle ear (ossicles) is the stirrup. The stirrup acts as doorman to the inner sanctum and advises the guards, but none of these three carries the sound wave in. The evidence for this radical departure from the traditional view is twofold. One point is that the gap between the anvil and stirrup is too large (up to 1mm) to transmit sound with the fidelity required for human hearing. The guards could not therefore whisper in the ear of the doorman – though the doorman has leverage on the guards, for the stirrup is joined to the anvil by cartilage. The other argument relates to the embryological origins of the parts in question. The stirrup's embryological source is completely different to that of the hammer and anvil. More recent research by Freeman[10] and Seaman[11] also suggests that a fluid pathway is at least as important as sound conduction through bone. It is now thought that vibrations of the skull bones may induce audio-frequency sound pressures in the skull contents, i.e. the brain and cerebro-spinal fluid. These vibrations are then thought to be communicated via liquid-like channels to the liquids of the inner ear.

Traditionally the ear is seen as being in three parts – outer, middle and inner – but Tomatis insists that it functions as two parts; inner

9   Thompson, B., 'Listening Disabilities: The Plight of Many,' in *Perspectives on Listening,* Wolvin, A. D; and Coakley, C. W., Ablex, New Jersey, 1993.

10 Freeman S; Sichel JY; Sohmer H., 'Bone conduction experiments in animals - evidence for a non-osseous mechanism,' *Hearing Research,* 146, 2000, pp.72-80. Cited on: http://onderwijs1.amc.nl/medfysica/doc/Bone%20conduction.htm

11 Seaman RL., 'Non-osseous sound transmission to the inner ear,' *Hearing Research,* 166, 2002, pp.214-215. Cited on: http://onderwijs1.amc.nl/medfysica/doc/Bone%20 conduction.htm

and outer, with the division being between the anvil and stirrup. This reflects the different origins as well as the different functions of these parts. The outer ear serves as a gatherer of sound information, while the internal ear, to which the stirrup belongs, is the organ of analysis. In other words, the Executive unit in the internal ear does the job of interpreting sound waves into a message that will mean something to the Director (the brain).

While the guards form a team with the receptionist, the doorman (the stirrup) acts only under the orders of its muscle (the stirrup muscle) which is the personal secretary to the Executive Team. These two are therefore party to the analysis and output of the Team's information. They make the decision, and inform the guards as to what visitors they will receive. The relevance of this fact is that, as a cortically-directed activity, listening is an active and volitional process, not a passive one. Sounds can only enter our neurological system with our consent.

The stirrup muscle is really a secretary extraordinaire for she never, ever rests. This is in fact the only muscle of the body which never rests. Even the heart, because it pulsates, is in effect taking intermittent rests, but the stirrup muscle is active from the fourth month in the womb until death. This continuous activity is required because the muscle plays a key role in cortical charge (in recharging the brain).

The inner ear

You, the visitor, the sound vibration, are now travelling through the mastoid bone, the bone which encases the inner ear. We have seen that it is not easy to reach the inner ear, which is deeply hidden and highly protected within the bone. The inner ear, called the cochlea, is a spiral shaped tunnel hollowed out of the mastoid bone, like the inside of a snail shell. The hearing organ itself, the organ of Corti, lies along the spiral shaped tunnel of the cochlea.

The whole chamber is filled with liquid. The fluid does not leave the chamber but its pressure is altered as needed by two flexible membranes, leading from the middle ear into the two main, parallel, spiral tunnels of cochlea. One is the oval window which receives pressure from the footplate of the stirrup bone. The other is the round window, which allows the release of pressure from vibrations occurring in the cochlea.

The actual hearing organ, the organ of Corti is what we are calling the Executive Team. The organ of Corti lies along the spirallic chamber of the inner ear. This organ is made up of the members of the Executive Team which are the cells of Corti. They are extremely sophisticated, each one knowing its role in the harmonic arrangement of their play. Each group of cells is tuned to a different frequency, so if it is destroyed, the ability to hear that frequency band is lost. However, in some cases the Corti cells have just been over-stressed by damaging noise. Any executive will break down under too much stress, but with the right kind of rehabilitation they can return to work. This is what the gentle stimulation of Sound Therapy appears to achieve for the Corti cells.

Each Corti cell bears 50 to 100 cilia – tiny hairlike cells like little antennae, sending and receiving signals as they vibrate within their liquid chamber. In total, the cochlea contains close to 30,000 of these cilia. The cilia are not passive receivers but active participants in the whole event, for the vibratory activity within the cochlea comes as much from cortical inputs from the brain as from external sound waves.

You – the travelling sound vibration – have arrived through the surrounding bone and entered the cochlea. You will find the Executive Team in a state of excitation – throbbing with its own information as it also receives and processes your message. Once it is processed, the message will be telephoned through to the Director who is not situated in the ear, but in the auditory cortex of the brain. The telephone system used for this final transmission is, of course, the auditory nerve, (the 8th cranial pair).

Interdepartmental connections

It is the job of the cortex then to organize and co-ordinate communication going back to the sensory organs, (eyes, ears, etc.) The eye perceives light and colour in the world by receiving different electromagnetic waves. The brain then makes sense of this information by instructing the eye to move and change its focus, using the oculomotor nerves. It is the brain that controls and directs the gaze in such a way that we can make sense of the incoming visual signals we receive.

The same process occurs in relation to the ear. The sound wave reaches the inner ear. The inner ear then transforms it into an electrochemical signal and the auditory nerve carries it to the cortex. This same auditory nerve brings back, to the inner ear, signals from the brain, which have been enhanced by input from many parts of the brain. In view of instructions received from the brain, the ear then adapts its way of attuning itself to the source of the sound. It is the desire and intention of the individual that therefore controls our willingness to listen.

So we can see that the whole organization of the ear is functioning at the discretion of, and under the intricate supervision of its Director, the brain. In order to competently orchestrate the process of hearing, the Director receives input from other departments and ensures the integration of their reporting systems. As an example, to listen with focus and purposefulness, the posture must be poised and balanced to have the whole body in an alert state. This occurs automatically, due to the way the inner ear is designed to work in total harmony with the vestibular system, which controls our posture and balance.

Checks and balance

Let us visit the vestibular system for it is in fact part of the ear, being continuous with the fluid-filled chamber of the cochlea. The vestibular system consists of three semi-circular canals. These contain sensors which tell us which way the head is tilted. The vestibular system is fed by the same nerve as the cochlea, and being part of the same pressure chamber, it is also regulated by the stirrup muscle. The stirrup muscle, therefore, according to Tomatis's theory, could be seen as the secretary to the Executive Team of balance as well as hearing. Therefore if this muscle is in spasm we will experience not only loss of hearing but dizzy spells as well.

Under the direction of the cortex, Tomatis maintains, the stirrup muscle controls and moderates strong vibrations, particularly those coming from our own voice. These self-generated sounds which we hear directly through bone conduction would be so loud, if not controlled, as to completely drown out the external sounds coming from our environment. So the stirrup's role is to dampen our inner bodily noises so that we can hear. It is not uncommon when people begin to lose their hearing, for them to be plagued by rumblings and pulsing generated from within the body. This indicates that the stirrup is losing its focus and the ear is unable to fulfill its function.

Some people may have experienced this effect when they had an ear infection. It can also be recreated to some extent if you block your ears and notice how your voice becomes loud and echoey because the external sounds are blocked off.

The stirrup muscle is supplied by the facial nerve (the 7th cranial pair) which is why facial expression is tied into our listening. The tensor tympani muscle of the hammer and anvil – guards of the receptionist – is supplied by the 5th or trigeminal nerve which also supplies the jaw. Movement of the jaw, of course, plays a part in equalizing air pressure in the middle ear and helping the ear drum to maintain its tonicity. Rigidity in the jaw also reflects our willingness, or lack of, to be open to incoming sounds. Cases of chronic jaw and neck tension can induce tinnitus, and nearly all tinnitus sufferers will acknowledge that their condition gets worse under stress.

The final relationship to be explored is that between the ear and the eye. The optic and oculomotor nerves, 2, 3, 4 and 6 are linked to eye, head and neck mobility. The co-ordinated interplay of these functions is, however, under the control of the acoustic nerve (8th nerve) responsible for hearing and balance. It is for this reason that while we listen we also turn our gaze in that direction; if we wear eyeglasses we reach for them when we concentrate on listening.

Sound Therapy and the ear

Now that we have the picture of what goes on inside the ear let us look at how Sound Therapy impacts on this system. Dr. Tomatis discovered that hearing acuity is not a static and unchangeable or steadily deteriorating function. It is an ever-changing set of complex relationships between ear, brain and psyche. He showed us how to access this system in order to improve the whole dynamic texture of our relationship with sound. Tomatis suggests that this means several things: that voice quality is enriched, hearing is improved, the ability to deal with language and communication leaps ahead and the brain is able to receive stimulating, recharging sounds.[12]

The first law of Tomatis is: "The voice contains only what the ear hears." He determined that if certain frequencies are missing from the hearing they will also be absent from the voice. Voice production is only possible through self-listening. If we cannot hear the sound we are producing, we fail to modulate and tune the voice, so we cannot of course reproduce frequencies we cannot hear.

His second law represents the change that is possible through using his method: "If the lost frequencies are restored to the hearing they will be automatically restored to the voice." The idea that hearing perception can be improved is ground-breaking, so let us look again inside the ear and see how this occurs.

As you know, the ear only admits sound if such a decision is approved by the Director and the Executive Team (the brain and the cochlea). But what if certain members of the organization are not performing their jobs properly? What if the ear has been bombarded for too

---

12   Tomatis, A.A., *The Conscious Ear*, Ibid.

many years by loud noise? Or what if an unconscious decision has been made to shut out the world? If the Director's team is not demanding a response from the organization, the organization falls into disarray and loses its ability to respond. A chain of disharmony descends from the Director, throughout the entire organization. What we find in these cases is poor tone in the middle ear muscles, the stirrup and hammer muscles. This means that the secretary and the guards are falling asleep on the job! So what is the receptionist to do? Without their guidance, the ear drum does not know how to respond to incoming sound.

First the Director needs a wake-up call, or perhaps a stimulating course in management. Sound Therapy provides this needed stimulation, building and reactivating the brain's potential. The lazy workers (ear muscles) are in need of physiotherapy. They need limbering up and waking up – so what better than an aerobics class? The constant fluctuation of high and low sound provided by the Electronic Ear within the complex rhythms and harmonies of classical music gets the ear muscles hopping, or rocking! However, the guards will only receive these gymnastic instructions if they come from the chief of the organization. It is the response of the brain to these interesting and stimulating sounds that in turn activates the ear muscles. This repeated activity re-sensitises them to the full range of sounds. The exercise program must of course be maintained regularly to get the muscles back in a fit state.

This brings us to the third law of Tomatis which is that: "Hearing which is compulsory, continual and repeated over a certain period of time definitely modifies hearing and speech." Dr. Tomatis found that in order for his therapy to have a lasting effect on improving the range of hearing, it must be used continuously for a certain period. The length of time varies depending on the individual and the severity of their problem.

Once the Sound Therapy program has taken effect, the Director is on the job, the guards are awake, the secretary is in full form and all messages are getting through efficiently to the Executive Team.

Sound vibrations reach the cochlea and if they are stimulating, charging sounds, such as Sound Therapy, the Corti cells become enlivened. While in response to the drone of an air conditioner or traffic noise these cells go into a dull and lifeless state, high frequency sounds re-awaken them. The hair-like cilia perk up and tremble with excitement as the waves of high harmonics dance up and down the organ of Corti. The ear is now playing its intended role of full alertness to incoming sound and of translating that sound, not only into meaning but into cortical charge.

Credits and debits

Concerning cortical charge, like a competent director we should always ask if the sound we are hearing is adding to or subtracting from our energy balance. Dr. Tomatis says that the ear's primary purpose is to provide a cortical charge in terms of electrical potential, but only certain sounds can achieve this charging effect. Low frequency sounds are a "debit" to the system while highs boost the credit balance. The Director, the conscious individual, decides where the body will go and to what sounds it will be exposed. The guards and secretary are fully at the call of the Director, so it is ultimately our brain, not our ear, that decides which sounds we will attend to. However, such attendance is only possible if our ear mechanisms are in good shape. A healthy organisation requires good judgment from an attentive management team and a healthy vibrant workforce to implement those decisions.

Although the world is full of noise hazards, we now have a choice. When we are forced to go into a noisy environment we can take Sound Therapy with us so that the effect of noise is being counteracted even as it happens.

Chapter Two

The Latest Developments and Applications for Sound Therapy

66 *As is well-known, sound has great power over inorganic* 99
matter. By means of sound it is possible to cause geometric
figures to form in sand and also to cause objects to be
shattered. How much more powerful, then, must be the
impact of this force on the vibrating, living substance of our
sensitive bodies.

Roberto Assigioli M.D.

Since 1984, when this book was first published, the role of sound as healer has gained much greater attention. A large amount of scientific research has proven the healing potential of music.[13] As thousands of people have been able to benefit from the self-help program we have realized that the scope of Sound Therapy is far larger than we imagined. In the years that I have been working with Sound Therapy people have told me that it improved their tennis, their driving, their singing and their sex life. One 80-year-old man even told me that, as a result of the therapy, he overcame his dizziness and was dancing down the street! Another man said it made such a difference to his health that he was getting married. One of my favourite testimonials was from a woman who said that the moment she put on the therapy she felt as though someone had placed a warm hand between two wet blankets in her brain.

In addition to being used by individuals on a search for self-improvement, the program has been used by many different

---

13 Hillecke, T. K; Nickel A. K; Bolay, H.V., 'Scientific Perspectives of Music Therapy,' *Annals of the New York Academy of Sciences*, 1060, 2005, pp.271-282.

professionals as an extension of their work. Remedial teachers, naturopaths, osteopaths, psychologists, speech pathologists, massage therapists, singing teachers, nurses, carers, and an increasing number of audiologists and medical doctors have introduced Sound Therapy into their practices. The self-help program is ideal for use by such practitioners because it is simple, compact, requires no special equipment, beyond a personal music player, and no special diagnostic testing. Any person working in a professional capacity with clients can easily incorporate Sound Therapy into their work. *The Practitioners Manual*, available from Sound Therapy International, gives a quick briefing to allow the professional to provide the necessary back-up information to support their clients in using Sound Therapy. A full Practitioner Education Program is also available by distance education and several hundred practitioners have undertaken this program to become Sound Therapy Consultants.

Professional applications

A number of teachers in special remedial classrooms have incorporated Sound Therapy with some success. In some instances the school purchased the program and allowed the children to use it for a period of time while at school. This meant, however, that listening time was limited for each child. A more thorough approach was where the school asked parents to purchase their own Sound Therapy program for their child. The child was then able to listen for much of the day while in class as well as having the albums to use at home.

Those teachers who were able to observe a number of children using the Sound Therapy were fully convinced of its benefits. All of the children showed some improvement; they became more settled in their behaviour, more communicative, and found it much easier to learn. One teacher told us of a little boy who had never been able to learn to spell: after Sound Therapy he began learning in leaps and bounds and said "I don't understand why it was so difficult before!"

The therapy helped children with ADD/ADHD, epilepsy, dyslexia, delayed speech and a wide range of learning difficulties. The results were comparative to those found in a variety of studies on the Tomatis method. [14, 15]

The Society for Brain Injured Children has recommended Sound Therapy to many families, as this is one of the few ways of directly stimulating the brain with an external input. It is a great complement to labour intensive therapies such as physiotherapy or speech therapy.

Body-workers of various types have introduced their clients to Sound Therapy. These include osteopaths, chiropractors, remedial massage therapists, yoga teachers, Feldenkrais practitioners and Alexander Technique teachers among others. Again, to get the full benefit of the program, clients need to purchase their own program and undertake regular listening. In some instances Sound Therapy brings about an immediate and dramatic change in neck tension and overall stress levels, rendering the body-work much more effective. Patrese Hosking, a body worker who has developed a unique method of improving spinal alignment and has over 40 years of clinical experience in her field, described how one of her first patients to use Sound Therapy came back for treatment after his first few days of listening. There was such a dramatic reduction in his neck tension that she was amazed, never having seen such a recovery before.

Naturopaths and medical doctors who are seeking additional ways to help their patients, recommend Sound Therapy as a treatment for stress, insomnia, tinnitus and other hearing difficulties. Combined with appropriate dietary changes and nutritional supplementation they have found Sound Therapy is of added benefit. Clive Tasker, N.D., former president of the Australian Natural Therapy

---

14 Madaule, Paul, *When Listening Comes Alive*, Moulin Publishing, Norval, Ontario, Canada, 1993.

15 Gilmor T.M., 'The efficacy of the Tomatis Method for children with learning and communication disorders: a Meta-analysis,' *International Journal of Listening*, 13, 1999, pp.12-23.

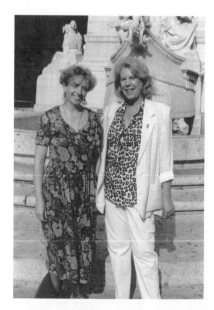

Rafaele Joudry and Lynn Schroeder – author of SuperLearning 2000 – *in New York*

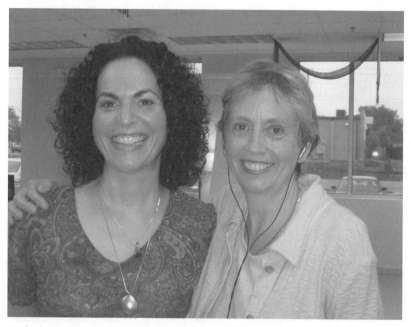

Rafaele Joudry and Dr. Donna Segal in Indianapolis 2006

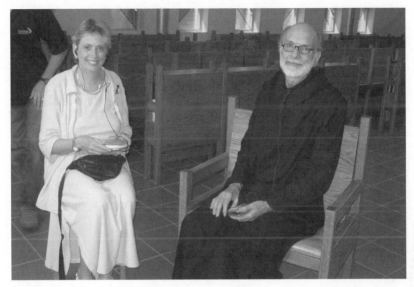

Rafaele Joudry interviewing Father Lawrence at St Peter's Abbey in 2006

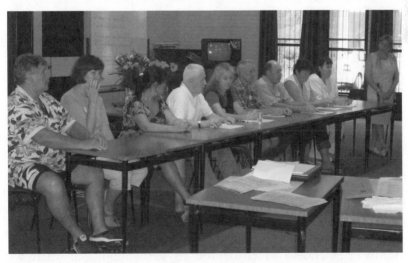

Practitioners panel at Sound Therapy Distributors Summit 2005

Association, also reported considerable success in using the program for tinnitus sufferers.

The Holistic Nurses Association is working towards the incorporation of natural therapies into medical practice. Many of their members have explored Sound Therapy as well as aromatherapy, reflexology and other natural approaches to healing.

Sound Therapy has come to the attention of many innovative researchers and health educators. Sheila Ostrander and Lynn Schroeder, in their groundbreaking book, *Superlearning 2000*, which brought accelerated learning into the mainstream, wrote the following:

> *"Father Lawrence's and Joudry's vision of the evolutionary powers of music to heal and rebalance began to become a reality for thousands... worldwide, do-it-yourselfers trying out this high frequency music were confirming what Lozanov and Bulgarian scientists had researched in secret so many decades ago: certain kinds of music, with very specific frequencies, harmonics, and complex structures, have startling powers to heal and empower us. And harnessing this music to the learning process is the route to evolutionary new mind powers. ... instead of having your mental powers deteriorate with age, your ear can become your antenna for life force. Stimulation has been shown to keep memory alive in the elderly."[16]*

In your own hands

Most of us rely on scientific, medical knowledge to look after our health and bring us the answers. We expect there to be a prescription for any ill. In the case of many chronic ear problems or difficulties of brain function, this is not always the case. Some of the conditions that Sound Therapy addresses are complex issues of health degeneration which require a systemic approach where we look at many aspects of our environment and lifestyle.

16 Ostrander, S. and Schroeder, L., *Superlearning 2000*, Dell, New York, 1994.

A large number of people have been affected by work-related noise, either in industry, agriculture, transportation, military service, entertainment or call center work. Many people seeking our help today spent most of their working life at a time when hearing protection was not the norm and was not available. Accumulated noise exposure over a period of many years frequently results in ear problems later in life.

Those working in call centers and entertainment industries may not have the option of using ear protection even today. Amplified and concentrated sound through headphones, experienced by radio presenters and call center operators, day in and day out, plus the occasional loud squeal from technical malfunctions, can be very damaging for some people.

Even more damage is probably done by younger individuals listening to music recreationally at concerts and on personal music players with earphones. The unfortunate habit of playing music at high volumes which are unsafe for the ear, frequently results in tinnitus, hearing loss and other ear problems later in life.[17]

As awareness of these dangers increases, more and more young people are wearing ear plugs to rock concerts and one day someone will think of turning down the volume! While we regulate the allowable levels of noise exposure in industry, there is no such safeguard for recreation. Industry standards allow exposure to 110 decibels for no more than one minute. However the sound level at rock concerts is commonly in the range of 90 to 130 decibels! Change will only happen consistently when recreational noise levels are legally controlled, which should be the role of the Environmental Protection Agency. In France and some other European countries the decibel level on personal music players must be limited by the manufacturer. Such steps are imperative to protect public health, since it is clearly part of human nature for young people to take risks

---

17 LePage, Eric L; and Murray, Narelle M., 'Latent cochlear damage in personal stereo users: a study based on click-evoked otoacoustic emissions,' *MJA*, 169, 1998, pp.588-592.

that will cause damage in the longer term, not realizing the reality of the error until their own body starts to degenerate, decades later.

How to protect your hearing

Avoiding excessive noise exposure is the single most important step to take in protecting our hearing. Once the damage has occurred, it is vitally important to avoid continued exposure as much as possible.

There are also other steps that can assist a degree of recovery. As one of the most nutrient rich organs of the body, the ear needs the right balance of minerals and nutrients to function well. The body also needs to be free of excess chemical pollutants and heavy metals, which can affect the nervous system, the musculo-skeletal system, the immune system and other bodily processes that impact on the ear.[18]

In the new, cutting edge field of environmental medicine, steps are taken to eliminate environmental toxins from both the body and the environment. Extra nutrients in the form of nutritional supplements may be used to help the body to rid itself of toxins and re-establish its correct equilibrium. Other environmental factors such as noise, stress and family and community support may need to be modified.

Auditory stimulation

The early introduction of hearing aids has been proven to assist in retaining and enhancing brain activity for sound processing. This is because the central auditory system of a person with hearing loss will experience deprivation-related plasticity. This means that physiological maps in the brain which are used to code frequency information will change when they have not been activated for a period of time.[19] For this reason it is wise to have a hearing aid

---

18 'Environmental Impact on Hearing: Is Anyone Listening?' *Environmental Health Perspectives,* Vol. 102, No.12, December 1994. Cited on 31 Aug 2009: http://www.ehponline.org/docs/1994/102-11/focus2.html
19 Tremblay, K. L., 'Hearing Aids and the Brain: What's the Connection?' *The Hearing Journal,* Vol.. 59, No. 8, August 2006, p.10.

fitted sooner rather than later. Increased auditory stimulation can be achieved with hearing aids, and this process will be further enhanced by the use of Sound Therapy.[20]

Other multi-sensory therapies can be used to assist greater brain integration, including bodywork, stress reduction, movement activities, and vision therapy. These therapies may be available through a range of allied health practitioners and clinics. Many of them are also available as self-help therapies, enabling you to take charge of your healing and have the solutions you need in your own hands.

Information and empowerment

There is a sense of personal empowerment that comes with managing your own healing, and learning to make your own choices about your health.

Increasing numbers of health-conscious individuals are using Sound Therapy to address damage caused by environmental noise and stress. By providing information including audio-visual and online support tools, Sound Therapy International aims to bring this sense of personal empowerment to the individual.

Like many other natural therapies, this puts individual people more in control of their own health. These therapies depend on the users becoming informed, learning to know their own bodies, being aware of the effects of the foods they eat, the sounds they hear and even the thoughts they think.

It's your life, your body, your ears, your planet, your choice. In this environment of personal empowerment, the self-help approach to Sound Therapy works perfectly. The program is in your hands, because once you are armed with basic information, no-one knows better than you do what your body needs.

---

20 Willott, J., 'Physiological Plasticity in the Auditory System and its Possible Relevance to Hearing Aid Use, Deprivation Effects, and Acclimatization,' *Ear and Hearing*, Vol.17, No.3, June 1996, pp.66S-77S.

The office environment

Sound Therapy is a perfect complement to the age of computers. More and more people are spending a large part of their lives in front of a computer, writing, researching, working from home, surfing the net. This is an ideal situation for using Sound Therapy. When working with a computer we are usually exposed to the low hum of the fan. This noise is tiring and draining for the brain. We are also exposed to radiation which tires the immune system.[21] It is easy to don your head-phones and listen to Sound Therapy while you are working on the computer. The gentle high frequencies provide stimulating and interesting sound to engage your auditory pathways as opposed to the monotonous and tiring sound of office equipment. Listeners have reported to us that as a result they finish a day's work rejuvenated and replenished instead of dragged out and weary.

People sometimes ask if they can use Sound Therapy when they work a lot on the phone. There are several ways to do this as long as you keep the volume low enough. You can leave the Sound Therapy in the right ear alone and hold the phone to the left ear or you can simply hold the phone on top of your mini earphone. You will be able to hear the person speaking over the music, just as you could if they were in the room with you. Or you can use a speaker phone, which doesn't interfere at all with wearing your Sound Therapy earphones.

Educational tools

As an education service we have developed various tools to help people understand Sound Therapy and to communicate the information to those who need it. Our educational DVD, *An Introduction to Sound Therapy*, contains interviews with several listeners who share their stories of successfully overcoming stress, epilepsy, travel fatigue,

---

21 Maisch, D; Rapley, B; Rowland, R.E; Podd, J., 'Chronic Fatigue Syndrome - Is prolonged exposure to environmental level powerline frequency electromagnetic fields a co-factor to consider in treatment?' *Journal of the Australasian College of Nutritional & Environmental Medicine*, Vol. 17, No. 2, December 1998, pp. 29-35.

tinnitus, hearing loss and learning difficulties. The DVD is a good tool for showing to self-help groups, parent groups or people who for any reason cannot read this book. Other DVDs provided with the program include lectures by those who have applied Sound Therapy for dementia, learning difficulties and improved ear and brain function.

For professionals, the *Practitioners Manual* provides the necessary background of research data, anatomical understanding and treatment suggestions to allow the incorporation of Sound Therapy into another type of practice.

Since 2002, in response to the public's need for more specific information, I have written two more books which explore particular applications for Sound Therapy. *Triumph Over Tinnitus* covers the topic of tinnitus in depth, including treatment with Sound Therapy and many other effective self-help methods. *Why Aren't I Learning?* is a book for parents and children's learning specialists. It explores the latest discoveries about auditory processing and sensory integration, explaining how Sound Therapy is relevant for a wide range of challenges facing children today, be it learning difficulties, dyslexia, ADHD, autism, or various other developmental issues. A more compact booklet called *Listening Helps Learning* serves as a brief instruction manual, providing all the necessary information to administer the program for children.

Over the course of two decades that we have been offering Sound Therapy programs to the public we have of course learned more about the effect of filtering algorithms on different conditions and how to best structure the Sound Therapy program for best results. We have made alterations to the filtering, the music selection and the listener support materials, adding to Tomatis's original processes and continuing to bring a better and better product to the public.

Chapter Three

What Sound Therapy Can Do for You. The results for specific conditions

66   *Music is a strange thing. I would almost say it is a miracle.*   99
For it stands half way between thought and phenomenon,
between spirit and matter, a sort of nebulous mediator, like
and unlike each of the things it mediates – spirit that requires
manifestation in time and matter that can do without space…
we do not know what music is.

Heinrich Heine

Rehabilitating the ear

Probably the three most common hearing problems in the community are hearing loss, tinnitus and difficulties in differentiating sound. The last condition may not show up on a hearing test, yet sufferers have such difficulty socialising in noisy environments that their social lives are often seriously curtailed. The name given to this condition by audiologists is "the cocktail party syndrome" or poor auditory discrimination.

Other fairly prevalent ear problems are dizziness, tiredness, atonal hearing, the inability to concentrate on what is being said by another (a condition which falls into the category of learning difficulties), hyperacusis (sound sensitivity) and speech problems associated with linear, sequential processing or reduced perception of certain frequencies.

Statistics gathered by Access Economics in 2006 indicate that over half the population aged 60 to 70 experience some form of hearing problem. After age 70 the likelihood increases to over 70 percent.[22]

The need for the brain to be stimulated by sound in order to maintain mental acuity and good energy levels also increases with age. Dr. Tomatis stated that the brain requires two billion stimuli per second for at least four hours a day in order to function at maximum potential.[23] Tomatis claimed that through prolonged exposure to noise, the ear gradually closes down, eliminating its ability to hear high frequencies. The brain is then starved of necessary stimulation leading to listlessness and low energy. This parallels the discovery of more recent research that the auditory deprivation from hearing loss results in changes in our brain maps, known as "deprivation related plasticity." [24] It is now also known that beneficial changes in plasticity can occur with sufficient stimulation, and Sound Therapy is aimed at creating this type of result. The famous American neurologist Oliver Sachs, whose achievements were highlighted in the movie *Awakenings* as well as his many books, has observed that music has the ability to move those who can't walk to dance, those who can't speak to sing and those who can't remember to remember.[25]

The older population

Sound Therapy may bring about a dramatic shift in energy levels and well-being and this is often most marked among the older population, who are the ones most in need of the energy lift and the re-opening of the ear to high frequencies. Due to the prolonged accumulation of the effects of noise, as well as the effects of ageing, older people are more likely to suffer from hearing disorders. Other health and mobility factors can also affect social interaction in later years, so it is particularly important to the older population to have intact hearing in order to maintain communication. Any degree

22 Access Economics, *Listen Hear: The Economic Impact and Cost of Hearing Loss in Australia,* CRC Hear and the Victorian Deaf Society, 2006.
23 Tomatis, A.A., *The Conscious Ear,* Ibid.
24 Tremblay, K. L., Ibid, p.10.
25 Ostrander, S. and Schroeder, L., Ibid.

of improvement to hearing or auditory discrimination can bring about a very meaningful difference in the social fulfillment of an older person. They have told us that Sound Therapy enables them to participate again in lunches at a restaurant or a bridge club, instead of having to constantly ask for things to be repeated or simply pretend to nod along but be left out of the real conversation.

Young people

More and more young people are realizing, from experience, the need for Sound Therapy. Sadly, due to the advent of amplified sound, a whole generation has suffered ear damage. The singer Fiona Horne, formerly lead singer with the band Deaf FX, contracted tinnitus, as many rock musicians do. She became a Sound Therapy listener and was enthusiastic about the relief she achieved through the program. Young people are wise if they take up listening as a preventive measure, just as people nowadays take up exercise programs to prevent heart trouble. Sound Therapy, combined with taking reasonable measures to avoid exposure to excessive noise, is the best insurance we have against the development of tinnitus or other hearing problems, in later life.

Tinnitus (ringing in the ears)

A 65-year-old man contacted us about his tinnitus. He had done a lot of rifle shooting when he was young and worked with chainsaws and farm equipment all his life. He was still driving a tractor for several hours a day, or working with other power tools.

He had had tinnitus, gradually worsening, for over 10 years. Early on he went to his doctor who told him that there was no treatment and he should learn to live with it.

On hearing of Sound Therapy, the man decided to give it a try as he had nothing to lose.

In the first two weeks he found he was sleeping better and much of the stress that came with tinnitus had lifted. He loved the serenity Sound Therapy gave him and enjoyed listening while driving the tractor and when going to sleep. There were times when the tinnitus seemed louder, but he understood that this was a normal part of the healing process.

After three months of Sound Therapy the tinnitus was greatly lessened, and after six months he hardly noticed it at all. During stressful times it increased a bit, but he was able to control it easily with Sound Therapy.

This is an example of a typical story, compiled from many of the tinnitus sufferers we have helped.

What is tinnitus?

Tinnitus is the condition where a phantom noise is heard inside the head. It may be continuous or intermittent, loud or soft. The sound can be anything from ringing to buzzing, hissing, rustling or roaring.

While some people are able to live with their tinnitus and ignore it most of the time, for others it can become a misery. It is sometimes hard for friends and loved ones to understand the stress, anxiety and exhaustion that can result from tinnitus.

Although it begins with a malfunction of the ear or the auditory system, other parts of the brain may become involved. The limbic system, which is the seat of emotions, may be stirred up by tinnitus, linking it to a state of alertness and anxiety.

The way we experience sound is that our neurons fire in certain parts of the brain, creating a pattern of brain activity that we experience as sound. When a person has tinnitus, the sound they hear internally is just as real to them as the sounds that come from outside. Both are experienced as neuronal firing, but one is caused from without and one from within.[26]

Tinnitus may be triggered by damage at any point along the auditory system. Beginning with the outer ear and the ear drum, this system also includes the middle ear, the inner ear, the auditory nerve and

---

26   Noble, B., 'Tinnitus and Clinical Psychology,' *Audinews*, 49(6/3) 2006.

the auditory cortex in the brain. (See Chapter 1 in Part 3, "Journey Through the Ear" for more detail on the anatomy of hearing.)

Some of the specific injuries or malfunctions commonly associated with tinnitus are:

- Damage to the sensory cells in the inner ear, which receive sound. One theory, "discordant theory" is that damage to these cells causes distortions in sound perception, which may result in tinnitus.[27]
- Faulty interaction "crosstalk" between the nerve fibres, for example the balance and the hearing nerve, caused by nerve compression.[28]
- Hyperactive brain cells, repeating a sense of sound stimulus when there is no external sound. This may be due to change in brain pathways in the auditory cortex or "plastic change."[29]
- Congestion or imbalance of fluid in the inner ear chambers, causing distortions in our perception of hearing.[30]

Specific factors which can cause tinnitus to develop are: exposure to excessively loud or prolonged noise, accidents causing injury to the ear or head, certain prescription drugs, ear infections and misalignment of the jaw. New information also indicates that an overload of chemical toxicity in the system and associated nutritional deficiencies could contribute to ear damage.[31]

When there is an injury or disturbance to any part of the auditory system, this may result in damage to the neural maps in parts of the brain responsible for hearing, and can sometimes lead to tinnitus.

---

27 Han, B.I; Lee, H.W; Kim, T.Y; Lim, J. S; and Shin, K.S., 'Tinnitus: Characteristics, Causes, Mechanisms, and Treatments,' *J. Clin. Neurol.*, 5(1) March 2009, pp.11–19. Published online March 31, 2009. doi: 10.3988/jcn.2009.5.1.11. PMCID: PMC2686891
28 Ibid.
29 Baguley, D. M; Humphriss, R. L; Axon, P.R; and Moffat, D. A., 'The Clinical Characteristics of Tinnitus in Patients with Vestibular Schwannoma,' *Skull Base*, 16(2) May 2006, pp.49–58.
30 Juhn, S.K; Hunder, B. A; Odland, R. M; 'Blood Labyrinth Barrier and Fluid Dynamics of the Inner Ear,' *Int. Tinnitus J.*, 7(2) 2001, pp.72-83.
31 'Environmental Impact on Hearing: Is Anyone Listening?' Ibid.

Tinnitus is now seen as the brain's response to a damaging or stressful impact on the hearing system.

Tinnitus recovery

The good news for tinnitus sufferers is that due to brain plasticity (the tendency of the brain to be constantly changing) the right sort of stimulation can correct this auditory mapping and increase our chances of restoring normal auditory functioning.

Until recently, the general medical belief was that tinnitus could not be treated, and the best strategy was to learn to live with it. This has prevented many people from seeking alternative tinnitus solutions. However, recent discoveries about brain plasticity have shown that recovery is possible from many types of brain disorders, including tinnitus, if the right sensory inputs and repetition of daily practices are used. Therefore, scientific opinion about the treatment of tinnitus is now changing.

Thousands of individuals, who were previously told to learn to live with their tinnitus, have turned to Sound Therapy, and many of those have been helped. My mother and I first became aware of tinnitus when people began writing to tell us their tinnitus had been cured or alleviated by Sound Therapy. We now have a thick file of letters from people who have experienced tinnitus relief through Sound Therapy. We have conducted several surveys of our listeners over the last twenty years and determined that between 80% to 90% of tinnitus sufferers benefited to some extent from Sound Therapy. I have also gone on to write another book about Sound Therapy and tinnitus, called *Triumph Over Tinnitus.*

Pulsatile tinnitus

In rare cases (about 3% of tinnitus patients) tinnitus will have a pulsing rhythm and seem to keep time with your pulse. This is called pulsatile tinnitus. These symptoms may indicate a vascular disorders such as a heart murmur, hardening of the arteries or hypertension. It is important to have these symptoms thoroughly investigated by your doctor or healthcare professional to find out the cause. These problems may be addressed through blood pressure medication or other medical interventions. Alternative treatments may also be available through a naturopath with nutritional supplementation and a change of diet. There have also been cases where Sound Therapy has provided additional relief with this type of tinnitus.

How can Sound Therapy help?

Sound Therapy impacts the entire auditory system, from the ear drum to the auditory cortex. Let's look at each part in turn as it relates to tinnitus. The middle ear (the air filled chamber behind the ear drum) contains two tiny muscles, the hammer and stirrup muscle, which play an active role in the functioning of the ear. Dr Tomatis theorised that the very subtle adjustment of these muscles is part of the process of the ear and brain being able to tune in or tune out to certain sounds. Lack of tone in these muscles therefore would mean that the ear would lose its ability to respond to certain frequency ranges, so these sounds never reach the inner ear. The ear's ability to adjust and balance the fluid pressure in the inner chambers is also impeded if the stirrup muscle is not fully functional.

These theories have yet to be scientifically tested, and research is needed in this area, but the results achieved by Sound Therapy listeners over many years does lend support to these ideas.

The Electronic Ear used in the recording of Sound Therapy challenges the human ear with constantly alternating sounds of high and low tone. At the same time, low frequency sounds are progressively removed from the music, so the ear is introduced to higher and higher frequencies. The resulting stimulation appears to bring about improvement in the functioning of the ear muscles, as it often reduces problems associated with the Eustachian tube, such as blocked ear.

What we think happens is that once the ear is able to recognize and admit high frequencies to the inner ear, the opportunity has been created for the hearing organ in the inner ear to be stimulated by the gentle and complex tones of Sound Therapy. It is possible that this music improves the function of the inner ear as well, though this mechanism is not yet fully understood.

What is now well established, by scientific research that has been done over the last couple of decades, is that music can stimulate the brain and alter the brain's response to sensory experience, and that this auditory remapping can assist with the reduction or elimination of tinnitus.

Vertigo and dizziness

Dizziness is a large-scale health issue, particularly among the older population. In a sample of people aged 65-75, one-third reported that dizziness and imbalance degraded the quality of their lives,[32] while balance-related falls account for more than one-half of the accidental deaths in the elderly. According to the NIH (National Institute of Health) in the US, 347,000 hospital days are incurred each year in the general population because of balance disorders.

Dizziness and vertigo relief through Sound Therapy

John Clancy, a music teacher, and founder of the Gippsland Chamber Opera Company, woke up one morning feeling dizzy. He also had a sense of liquid flooding the inside of his head and dry, sore eyes. These peculiar symptoms plagued him for eight months during which time he consulted no less than six general practitioners, two ear specialists, a physician, a neurologist, a chiropractor, an acupuncturist, a shiatsu masseur, a naturopath and a Chinese medical practitioner. None of them was able to help. While eye drops fixed the dry eyes, the ear problems proved a mystery because the doctors who examined him could find no problem with his ears – the organ of balance.

After a year, the dizzy sensations changed and he felt as though he was being pulled to the left. "It was on a trip to South America that I began to notice a few persistent patterns," said Clancy, describing

---

32   'A Report of the Task Force on the National Strategic Research Plan,' National Institute on Deafness and other Communication Disorders, National Institutes of Health, Bethesda, Maryland, April 1989, p.74.

how journeys by boat always produced attacks of imbalance. "A two hour crossing by boat from Colonia in Uruguay to Buenos Aires produced a severe attack which lasted for about three days." However he was puzzled that on a trek on the Inca Trail, at an altitude of about twelve thousand feet, the condition seemed to disappear.

The fact that this condition was alleviated at high altitude points clearly to a relationship between balance and air pressure. A reduction in air pressure at high altitude will also reduce the air pressure in the middle ear and may, in turn, impact the fluid pressure in the inner ear.

Clancy eventually decided to try Sound Therapy, since nothing else had given any promise of relief. This is what he had to say about Sound Therapy:

> *"For the first two or three weeks, I did not feel that any change was taking place. Then gradually I began to notice an improvement. The pull to the left side of my head seemed to be waning. My feelings of imbalance began to improve. I persisted with the therapy, confident now that things were under repair. I continued the Sound Therapy for the required three months. My sense of balance has now virtually returned to normal."*

How our sense of balance works

The role of the vestibular apparatus, (the semicircular canals in the inner ear) is to communicate to the brain, via the vestibular branch of the auditory nerve, that there is sudden movement of the head. When this sensation persists in the absence of real movement, it gives the patient the feeling that the world is spinning or falling away beneath them, as in a Meniere's attack.

There are several diagnoses which may be given for ear-related balance problems, including Meniere's syndrome, vestibular inflammation (neuronitis or labyrinthitis) or BPPV (Benign Paroxysmal Positional Vertigo.) If it is not ear-related, dizziness could be due to low blood pressure or a series of strokes affecting the parts of the brain which process our sense of balance.

Sound Therapy has proved helpful in many types of balance disorders and this could be for a number of reasons. Most notably:

1. Getting the middle ear muscles to relax may help to reduce excess pressure, fluid imbalances and inflammation of the inner ear mechanisms.[33]

2. The positive stimulation of the auditory pathways in the brain may help sensory integration and improve the way the brain provides our sense of balance through its interpretation of signals received from the eyes, ears and joint receptors.[34]

Meniere's

Meniere's syndrome is a diagnosis given to a set of symptoms which includes sudden dizzy attacks, low frequency tinnitus, a feeling of fullness in the ear, and progressive hearing loss. While the cause is unknown, there is evidence that the condition is related to too much pressure on one of the fluids in the inner ear. This fluid is called endolymph, and it is held in part of the cochlear spiral, called the scala media, as well as in the semi-circular canals which give us our sense of balance. The processes that occur in the inner ear are extremely complex and much of its workings are still not fully understood.

However several clinicians have observed that levels of fluid pressure in the whole body affect the pressure in the ear. For some women, dizzy attacks are more prevalent during the half of their

---

33 Klockhoff, I., 'Impedance fluctuation and a "tensor tympani" syndrome,' in: *Proceedings of 4th International Symposium on Acoustic Impedance Measurements,* edited by Penha and Pizarro,Universidade Nove de Lisboa, 1981, pp.69-76. Facsimile on www. tinnitus.org
Hazel, J., 'Things that go Bump in the Night,' from *ITHS Newsletter,* 5 Jan 2003.
Golz A; Fradis M; Martzu D; Netzer A; and Joachims HZ., 'Stapedius muscle myoclonus,' *Ann. Otol. Rhinol. Laryngol.,* 112(6) 2003, pp.522-4. Cited on: http://www.dizziness-and-balance.com/disorders/hearing/tinnitus.htm
34 Jones, E. G; and Powell, T. P. S., 'An Anatomical Study of Converging Sensory Pathways Within The Cerebral Cortex of the Monkey,' *Brain* 93, 1970, pp.793-820.

menstrual cycle prior to menstruation (from ovulation through the menstrual bleed). When fluid retention is relieved from the body after menstruation, it appears that this also reduces the pressure on the ear.[35]

Symptom management is typically achieved through the drug Serc. While this has been a life-saver for many people, it can have side effects with prolonged use. Meniere's is also often managed via the practice of reducing salt intake, to reduce fluid retention in the body, and this is found to help alleviate the dizziness.

However we need salt to help the body perform a variety of essential functions. Salt helps maintain the fluid in our blood cells and is used to transmit information in our nerves and muscles. It is also used in the uptake of certain nutrients from our small intestines. The body cannot make salt and so we are reliant on food to ensure that we get the required intake. Therefore it may be preferable to find another solution to Meniere's, rather than permanently going without an important mineral.

While we know that reducing fluid retention by cutting out salt does help to manage the symptoms of Meniere's, this does not explain why the dizzy attacks are typically so sudden. Dr. Tomatis has proposed that Meniere's's vertigo is due to an anomaly in the tension of the stirrup muscle in the middle ear.[36] This muscle may be subject to involuntary twitches or spasms, like any other muscle in the body. Such twitching would radically alter the fluid pressure in the inner ear chambers, thus causing havoc with the balance mechanism.

It may be due to the re-toning of the stirrup muscle achieved by Sound Therapy that listening helps to reduce or eliminate the dizzy attacks for some people. Research is needed in this area to determine how this mechanism occurs, and to clarify its relationship to Sound Therapy.

---

35 Morse, Dr. Gwen, 'Changes in Meniere's Disease Responses as a Function of the Menstrual Cycle,' cited on 9th August 2009, http://oto2.wustl.edu/men/mn8.htm
36 Tomatis, A.A., *The Conscious Ear*, Ibid.

In order to maintain good ear health and pressure regulation, we recommend that Meniere's sufferers continue long-term Sound Therapy listening. Though we do not fully understand the mechanism or progression of Meniere's, the improvement that some listeners have had with their dizziness shows that Sound Therapy increases healthy ear function, so we can surmise that long-term input may increase the chances of reducing degeneration.

Here is what one listener said about Meniere's:

> *"I've had Meniere's on and off for about ten years, I used to get so giddy I would have to call a doctor. It had become progressively worse, and I'd have an attack about once a fortnight. My attacks made me nauseous, and I'd get diarrhoea with it. If an attack happened at night, my husband had to take me to hospital for a shot of stematil or maxilon. I tried SERC, multi B forte and changed my diet, with little improvement.*
>
> *I started listening to Sound Therapy for three hours a day, and it was about eight weeks before I noticed a difference. I became able go up to three months without an attack or feeling giddy, and I've only had to have one shot in the last year, when I cut back to two hours listening a day. I'm back up to three hours a day listening now and I can't speak highly enough of it, Sound Therapy is a miracle for me, to change such a debilitating thing."*
>
> Name withheld.

Another said:

> *"So far the therapy has completely eliminated my attacks of Meniere's Syndrome. – a miracle."*
>
> Rupert Francis, Lower Templeston.

Another listener, Shirley Cowburn, shared her story on balance recovery in our very first edition of this book. Recently (i.e. now in 2009) she made contact again and wrote:

"I went to work, shopped, did housework and cooking at home and generally 'lived' with the earphones in my ears (a strange sight for a middle-aged woman in 1984!!) I only listened with the music in the background, not loudly at all. After about three months or so my balance, which had been awful for many years had gone back to normal. That was 25 years ago and I'm still the same today."

BPPV (Benign Paroxysmal Positional Vertigo)

Benign Paroxysmal Positional Vertigo (BPPV) is sometimes mistaken for Meniere's Disease and some people may receive both diagnoses from different practitioners. BPPV is generally typified by dizziness that comes on as a result of a particular movement: for example rolling over in bed, or bending to do up your shoes. BPPV can have many causes, and not all of them are well understood at this time. A popular current theory is that BPPV is usually caused by free-floating calcium crystals in the posterior semicircular canal, one of the three canals of the vestibular system.[37] There is a treatment, called the Epley manoeuvre, or canolith repositioning, in which the head is tilted in a certain procedure, by a trained practitioner, in order to dislodge the crystals from the canal. This may be effective temporarily or permanently. The audiologist or hearing clinic will help you to find a practitioner who knows how to do this manoeuvre. While it is usually done by a practitioner who has been trained in the procedure, it is easy enough so that doctors often teach it to BPPV sufferers and their families.

Because BPPV is a complex condition, possibly also involving the integration of sensory pathways in the brain, canolith repositioning may or may not provide a permanent solution. Some of those diagnosed with BPPV have also benefited from Sound Therapy,

---

37 Froehling DA; Bowen JM; et al., 'The canalith repositioning procedure for the treatment of benign paroxysmal positional vertigo: a randomized controlled trial,' Mayo Clinic Proceedings, 75(7) 2000, pp.695-700. Cited on 9th August 2009, from *Vertigo: Its Causes and Treatment*, Huai Y. Cheng, M.D.,
http://www.thedoctorwillseeyounow.com/articles/other/vertigo_17/

perhaps because it seems to improve the pressure balance in the ear and the transmission of signals between the ear and the brain.

Dizziness and the brain

We cannot separate ear function from the auditory pathways in the brain, because the way the brain processes sensory information from the eyes, joints and ears also creates our sense of balance. When this process is not occurring correctly, chronic vestibular integration disorder may result.

An example of a person suffering from a chronic vestibular integration disorder was Jeanette McKay, who lived constantly with a sense that the earth was moving beneath her feet. She had a lot of car sickness and other balance problems, and found this made everything in the way of learning much more difficult. In her own words, "I always felt the ground was moving, as if I was walking on a waterbed or something unstable. I didn't know that other people didn't experience this. Riding in a car I would have to watch the road all the time, even as a passenger. If anyone took a sharp turn or changed directions quickly while driving, it would really throw me out and make me feel ill, so I realised that I must have a problem with my vestibular system."

After she started using Sound Therapy Jeanette said, "I felt as though the earth was stable for the first time in my life." She added that, "after Sound Therapy, when that sense of constant motion stopped, I straight away felt more confident because I was more secure in my own body. It was the most amazing feeling. It also changed my peripheral vision and I believe part of that was the vestibular system settling down. I noticed that I had better depth perception, so instead of seeing everything as flat, I could see in 3D – depth was added to my world!"

By offering an integrated approach for the ear and brain pathways, Sound Therapy presents a totally different approach to the treatment of balance difficulties than any previously available.

Drug treatment for dizziness

Some doctors prescribe drugs called vestibular suppressants. These drugs can have unwanted side effects, such as lethargy and impaired balance, and the elderly are particularly sensitive to these side effects. For this reason they are given sparingly and only for more severe and long-lasting attacks.[38]

In contrast, Sound Therapy aims at enhancing connections between the vestibular system and sensory processing in the brain, potentially giving a natural and more permanent solution.

It is always better to solve these problems by addressing the cause within the body rather than by trying to control it with medication. There is evidence now, from the field of learning difficulties and sensory integration dysfunction, that some recovery is possible from sensory integration disorders, if we are just able to give the right stimulus to the brain, providing input via the muscles and sensory systems.[39]

If Sound Therapy can in fact produce improved balance, as some of our listeners have testified, it may be very beneficial for it to be used more widely, not just for sufferers of Meniere's or other specific balance disorders, but for the older population where a slight improvement to balance can make the difference between falling or not falling. An improvement in balance could potentially save a lot of injury and loss of independence for those living alone.

Hearing loss

Why does hearing deteriorate?

There are many contributing causes to hearing deterioration. Some of the more common ones are:

- Inner ear damage due to prolonged exposure to loud noise[40]

---

38 Ibid.
39 Kranowitz, C. S., *The Out of Synch Child,* Penguin, New York, 1998.
40 Access Economics, Ibid.

- Lack of high frequency sound to stimulate the ear [41]
- Ear damage or lack of good muscle tone in the middle ear, caused by stress, noise, injury, nutritional deficiency or repeated infections[42]
- Psychological factors – closing off to some frequencies due to psychological blocks or traumas, leading to inefficient processing of sound by the brain [43]
- Otosclerosis – caused by overgrowth of the cochlear bone, possibly caused by a mineral deficiency, which results in the fusion of the stirrup bone to the cochlea.[44]

Is deterioration inevitable with age?

We often assume that certain faculties must deteriorate with age, simply because we see this happening so often. However, recent brain research is showing us that the brain can regenerate more than we thought, if given the right stimulation and nutrition. The same is true for our sensory pathways.

To some degree, deterioration can be avoided. It is not the number of years of living that causes hearing damage, it is the number of years of noise abuse, poor diet and the impact on our health of exposure to environmental toxins. Young people who listen to rock music have a hearing level equal to fifty-year-old factory workers.[45]

However, some individuals, even those in their eighties have experienced noticeable improvement in their hearing through using Sound Therapy.

41 Moore, D. R; Rothholtz, V; and King, A. J., 'Hearing: Cortical Activation Does Matter,' *Current Biology*, Vol. 11, No.19, 2001, pp.R782-R784.
42 Klockhoff, I, Ibid.
43 Tomatis, *The Conscious Ear,* Ibid.
44 Minor, L. B., et al., 'Dehiscence of Bone Overlying the Superior Canal as a Cause of Apparent Conductive Hearing Loss,' *Otology & Neurotology*, Vol. 24, No. 2, March 2003, pp.270-278.
45 LePage, Eric L; and Murray, Narelle M., Ibid, pp.588-592.

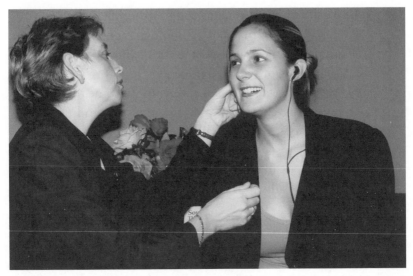

Rafaele Joudry helping a client with headphones

Sound Therapy and hearing aids

Sound Therapy should not be considered a replacement for hearing aids, but a tool that can help the ear and brain be more responsive, so in most cases the person can adjust more successfully to using a hearing aid. To adapt to a hearing aid requires retraining of the auditory system so that sound can be perceived accurately through this new technology. This adjustment requires the building of new maps or pathways in the brain, and such remapping can be enhanced by auditory stimulation, particularly that of Sound Therapy.

Different types of hearing loss

There are two types of hearing loss: conductive and sensorineural. Conductive hearing loss refers to any problems in the middle ear which prevent sound from being conducted to the inner ear. The more common type, sensorineural hearing loss, affects the inner ear and nervous system. The experience of hearing loss is then further compounded by the degeneration of auditory neural pathways, which occurs when there is a lack of auditory stimulation.

Conductive hearing loss

Conductive hearing loss occurs when there is a disorder in the sound transmission system in the middle ear. This includes Eustachian tube problems (recurrent blocked ear,) fluid or infections in the middle ear, or otosclerosis in which the bones of the middle ear become porous or calcified.

Otosclerosis is a condition said to affect 3% of the population. An overgrowth of the inner ear bones, causes the stapes (stirrup) bone in the middle ear to become fixed, so the middle ear loses its movement. There is a clear association between otosclerosis and osteoporosis (thinning of the bones). In its early stages otosclerosis is characterised by softening or sponginess of the ear bones. It is known to worsen after pregnancy, when women are also at greater risk of osteoporosis due to calcium depletion and hormone disruption. Therefore adequate calcium supplementation may be advisable to assist in the prevention of otosclerosis.[46]

Otosclerosis can sometimes be successfully corrected by surgery, and this may be the best option for severe cases. The operation, called a stapedectomy, usually involves replacing the stirrup bone with a prosthesis. To improve the success of the operation it can also be useful, both before and after the procedure, to use Sound Therapy. Bringing movement and flexibility to the ear muscles may improve circulation to the ear, assisting it to prepare for and recover from surgery, as physiotherapy is generally important after surgery. Sound Therapy is, according to Dr Tomatis, like physiotherapy for the ear.[47]

---

46 Clayton A.E. et al, 'Association between osteoporosis and otosclerosis in women,' *Journal of Laryngology & Otology* (2004), Vol.118, No.8, Royal Society of Medicine Press, pp.617-621.
De Chicchisa, E. R. et al, 'Vitamin D and calcium deficiency initiated in pregnancy and maintained after weaning accelerate auditory dysfunction in the offspring in BALB/cJ mice,' *Nutrition Research,* Vol. 26, No. 9, September 2006, pp.486-491.
Shambaugh GE Jr., 'The diagnosis and treatment of active cochlear otosclerosis,' *J Laryngol Otol.,* Vol. 85, 1971, pp.301-314. Cited 13th August 2009 on http://www.dizziness-and-balance.com/disorders/hearing/otoscler.html
47 Tomatis, *The Conscious Ear,* Ibid.

Sound Therapy, in combination with nutritional supplementation, has also been noted to improve hearing even when the patient does not opt for surgery. Narelle Russell, a farmer and mother of three children, experienced hearing degeneration from childhood. Her hearing became noticeably worse after each pregnancy and she was diagnosed with otosclerosis. As calcium in the body is depleted by pregnancy, this condition may worsen. She embarked on Sound Therapy listening and used the program for five years with great success, improving her hearing and reducing her tinnitus. When she added supplementation with colloidal minerals and antioxidants she found that her hearing actually improved, in spite of the otosclerosis.[48]

Some women have been successful in reversing osteoporosis with natural hormone balancing cream derived from wild yam and chaste tree berry.[49] An Italian grandmother, Cesaria Carpitano, aged in her 80s had degenerative osteoporosis and was walking with two sticks and in constant pain. After a few months of using the wild yam cream and high-quality mineral supplementation her bone density improved by 8.1%. She discarded her sticks and walked upright and pain-free.[50]

Excess tension or lack of tone in the middle ear muscles (hammer and stirrup muscle) may be a factor in some types of conductive hearing loss.[51] It appears that this tone may be restored through the exercise provided by Sound Therapy, and this has been observed to improve hearing in some cases of conductive hearing loss. [52]

---

48   Private conversations and video interview with Narelle Russell, Narooma, 2001-2006.
49   Shealy, C. N. *Natural Progesterone Cream, Safe and Natural Hormone Replacement,* Keats, Lincolnwood, Illinois, 1999.
50   Private conversations with Cusumano Family, Sydney 2000 – 2009.
51   http://en.wikipedia.org/wiki/Tensor_tympani
      This theory of Tomatis' that the tone and function of the middle ear muscles plays a role in hearing has not yet been explored by science, though a number of researchers have identified chronic conditions called 'tonic tensor tympani syndrome' which represent an extreme level of stapedial dysfunction. Research is needed on the more subtle effects of muscular performance and potential rehabilitation.
52   Tomatis, *The Conscious Ear,* Ibid.

Sensorineural hearing loss

Sensorineural hearing loss results from damage within the inner ear or cochlea itself, where the sensory cells transmit sound to the auditory nerve. Loud or prolonged noise damages the sensory cells – called cilia – in the inner ear. When the cilia are damaged or destroyed, they can no longer pick up sound vibrations, so the sound does not reach the auditory nerve. Other lifestyle factors or environmental toxins, including chemicals found in the home, or certain medications can also damage the cilia.[53] This condition is sometimes referred to as nerve deafness.

Auditory deprivation

Another mechanism that may compound the experience of hearing loss is a breakdown in communication between the ear and brain. This occurs when brain pathways required for hearing are not firing normally.

To combat this degeneration it is very important to provide stimulation to help keep the auditory pathways firing. Using a hearing aid will help to increase auditory stimulation, and research has shown that starting early is important so as not to leave the brain without that needed stimulation. We now know, from research in the field of brain plasticity, that by providing sufficient stimulation, new brain pathways can be built so that even when damage has occurred, the brain can learn new ways of responding to stimuli.[54]

Another way to increase stimulation to the auditory pathways is with Sound Therapy, which provides sound that is specifically tailored for activating the organ of hearing in the inner ear and associated brain pathways. Sound Therapy can be used with or without a hearing aid, and many listeners have found a noticeable improvement in their ability to hear, pay attention and understand voices in different environments and social situations.

---

53   Access Economics, Ibid.
     'Environmental Impact on Hearing: Is Anyone Listening?' Ibid.
54   Doige, N., Ibid

How does Sound Therapy help hearing?

In summary, Sound Therapy may help with the perception of hearing in several ways.

1. Auditory remapping

The brain is plastic, meaning its pathways can be changed or remapped with the right stimulation. To best maintain our hearing perception we need to practice actively listening and to receive sufficient stimulation of the right kind of sound to the auditory system.[55]

2. Exercising the middle ear muscles, hammer and stirrup muscles

Good muscle tone and flexibility are believed to be important for the fine tuning of the middle ear mechanism if it is to conduct sound accurately to the inner ear. The recording process used to make Sound Therapy albums presents the ear with alternating high and low tones, providing a dynamic stimulus to increase the tonicity of these muscles by causing them to repeatedly tense and relax. This is believed to reduce spasms and chronic tension which may prevent the muscles from doing their job.[56]

3. Stimulating the cilia

On the Sound Therapy albums the low frequency (low tone) sounds are progressively removed and the high frequencies are augmented. Although quiet, the high frequency sounds are raised in pitch until the predominant sounds heard are between 8,000 Hz and 16,000

---

55 Moore, D.R., Ibid.
56 While this is a new and fairly undeveloped field of research, investigations into "acoustic shock" (the condition where muscle spasms become permanent following dramatic acoustic events,) has evidenced that the functionality of these muscles does affect our ability to hear.
    Klockhoff, I., Ibid, pp.69-76.
    Ramírez, et al. 2007, 'Tensor Tympani Muscle: Strange Chewing Muscle,' *Med. Oral. Patol. Oral Cir. Bucal,* Vol.12, pp.96-100.
    Golz A; Fradis M; Martzu D; Netzer A; and Joachims HZ., Ibid. pp.522-4.

Hz. These high frequency sounds provide gentle but concentrated stimulation for the cilia and nerve pathways. Whether in fact this results in improved cochlear function has not been scientifically tested, but some Sound Therapy listeners do report a sense of improved hearing in the high frequencies. (See part 2 "Listeners Stories.")

4. Psychological opening

Hearing is sometimes closed down to some extent for psychological reasons. Tomatis held that Sound Therapy encourages resolution of psychological issues by re-introducing high frequency sound and re-creating the pre-birth experience of sound. As the psychological issues are resolved, the person may become more open to the full range of hearing. This also parallels the process of auditory remapping, in which new connections may be built between various parts of the brain.[57]

How effective is Sound Therapy for hearing loss?

More research is needed to determine the effectiveness of Sound Therapy on hearing loss. However, feedback received from Sound Therapy listeners over the last twenty years indicates that a variety of people experience some improvement in their hearing, and many have reported that as a result of Sound Therapy:

- their families no longer have to shout at them
- they can hear the birds again
- they can follow a group conversation
- the sounds are clearer and crisper
- they have more success in using and adjusting to their hearing aids.

Those people who have reported these benefits include: people with industrial deafness, people who were using a hearing aid 80% of the time, people in their eighties and people diagnosed with a wide variety of hearing-related disorders.

---

57 Tomatis *The Conscious Ear,* Ibid.

In our initial listener surveys, between 36% and 56% of respondents reported some noticeable hearing improvement. In some cases it requires several months of listening to improve hearing, so persistence is essential. The exact mechanism for this improvement is not yet known, but we feel confident in suggesting that the addition of Sound Therapy for those considering or using hearing aids, is likely to be beneficial both at the stage of adapting to the hearing aid and in the longer-term.

Blocked ear

Blocked ear is something we all experience when we have a cold or ear infection. Mucous and fluid builds up in the middle ear and Eustachian tube so that the ear cannot equalize. The fluid and the resulting air trap prevents the eardrum from vibrating freely, and this is why you feel deaf when you have a blocked ear. Some individuals suffer from chronic blocked ear which will not go away. Others may have frequent clicking and popping in the ears or have difficulty equalizing the ears when they ascend a mountain or fly in an aeroplane. This is due to some form of Eustachian tube malfunction, where the Eustachian tube is unable to open normally to allow the equalization of air pressure.

Four tiny muscles are responsible for the opening and closing of the Eustachian tube.[58, 59] One of them is a branch of the hammer muscle in the middle ear.[60] In cases of chronic Eustachian tube dysfunction, my theory is that in some cases this is due to a lack of tone and poor functioning of the Eustachian tube muscles. I suggest that Tomatis's theory that Sound Therapy rehabilitates the middle ear muscles[61] may also extend to the Eustachian tube muscles. This would explain why some Sound Therapy users who have chronic blocked ear have found relief for this condition after using Sound

---

58 Kuppersmith, R. B., 'Eustachian tube function and dysfunction,' July 11, 1996, cited on 13th Sept 2009. http://www.bcm.edu/oto/grand/71196.html
59 Gray, H. *Gray's Anatomy*, Fifteenth edition, Barnes and Noble, USA, 1995.
60 Gibson, Prof B., private conversation.
61 Weeks, Bradford S., Ibid, see Appendix 2.

Therapy. One such user, Katy Fitzgerald, was featured in an article in the *Sydney Morning Herald*. Here is an excerpt from the article:

'After treatment from several ear specialists, homeopathy and even ear ventilation tubes failed, Fitzgerald heard about Sound Therapy from her GP. ... Fitzgerald says the treatment has ended a lifetime of frustration. "It's made a really big difference for me. I always had good hearing but just had this echo. Now I can feel comfortable singing again."' [62]

Stress and energy

Stress is what happens when fear or anxiety becomes a constant state. The psychological effects include contracted muscles, increased heart rate and constricted breathing. The adrenal system is overtaxed and blood pressure rises. Stress interferes with the body's natural flow of energy. It cuts down our available energy and forces us to function on adrenaline.

Our energy level is determined by the functioning of chemical systems and nerve impulses throughout the body. Neural activity (the passage of information along our nerves) resembles electricity in several ways. The potential for excitation of the nerve synapses depends on the level of energy charge in the brain. Dr. Tomatis argued that the most important function of the ear is to recharge the brain through the stimulation of sound. Failure of the ear to provide sufficient recharge to the brain results in fatigue and inefficient mental processes.

Ninety percent of people suffer from low energy and stress overload. For all except those living in exceptional wilderness settings, noise plays a major part in their stress levels. The effect of Sound Therapy for the majority of people is to give a built-in defence against the effects of noise-induced stress.

---

62 Creagh, S., 'Why I use sound therapy,' *Sydney Morning Herald*, October 14, 2004.
    http://www.smh.com.au/articles/2004/10/14/1097607348327.html?from=moreStories

Noise

Normally we are not conscious of the role that noise plays in our stress levels, yet noise is one of the biggest contributors to stress and fatigue. Because the ear is directly linked by nerve paths to many other body organs, the sounds we hear have an immediate effect on our whole system. It is the high frequency sounds which replenish the brain's energy and activate the cortex, improving our ability to think. Unfortunately most of the sounds we hear in our mechanized, urbanized lifestyle are low frequency sounds. Sound Therapy offers the opportunity to listen to healing, high frequency sounds even in the midst of a busy, noisy environment.

Brain activity is always either enhanced or depleted by sound, depending on the quality of the sound. This is why Dr. Tomatis said, "Some sounds are as good as two cups of coffee." Listening to these albums for three hours a day compensates for and counteracts the draining, stressful effect of low frequency noise.

Of course, where there are other debilitating factors such as chronic disease or chemical overload, other approaches such as looking at diet, exercise and nutritional supplementation may also be necessary, but Sound Therapy provides one major and frequently overlooked piece of the puzzle.

Sleep

The purpose of sleep is to replenish the brain's energy. Dr. Tomatis's discovery has shown that if we receive sufficient stimulation for the brain, the need for sleep is reduced. Studies have found that deep sleep, medically termed "hypersomnia", is the most essential type of sleep for our well-being. Dreaming sleep, or REM (Rapid Eye Movement) is a lighter sleep, and if the brain receives adequate stimulation from Sound Therapy, it can be reduced in length without ill effects.

A Sound Therapy listener does not accumulate tiredness during the day but has an energized tranquillity that enables rest. The therapy improves the quality of sleep, usually producing a profoundly restful slumber even for people who have been restless sleepers. Through gaining deeper sleep, many listeners find that they need less sleep and can reduce their requirements by two to three hours per night. Dreams are often changed, nightmares subside and clear, positive dreams are recalled.

Insomnia

Insomnia is caused by excessive cortical activity that cannot be stopped. Though Sound Therapy recharges the brain for activity during the day, it also has a calming effect which enables the listener in nearly every case to slip easily and quickly into sleep. While the brain and the nervous system are stimulated by the sound, this results not in a hyperactive state but in a state of active serenity, which allows for deep rest. Sleeplessness due to anxiety can also be resolved.

Survey results indicate that between 70 and 80 percent of Sound Therapy listeners notice an improvement in their sleep. Many insomniacs experience an immediate and dramatic improvement in their sleep.

Communication

When hearing is impaired, speech is also affected. The voice cannot produce sounds that we cannot hear, because self-listening is integral to voice production. Therefore when hearing is impaired the voice becomes monotone and lifeless, lacking the qualities to inspire active listening in others. As Sound Therapy repairs distortions in the listening curve, the range and quality of the voice is enhanced.

Stuttering is another failure of the listening cycle. Tomatis describes the fascinating series of discoveries he made with singers, dyslexics and stutterers, leading to his conclusion that right ear dominance produces more efficient auditory processing. He theorizes that poor lateralization, meaning the co-ordination of the right and left ears with the cerebral hemispheres, causes a delay in the speaking and self-listening cycle. A transcerebral delay time in the order of .15

seconds will result in a stutter, he says.[63] Sound Therapy aims to encourage right laterality by feeding more sound to the right ear.

The right ear, as opposed to the left, is more directly linked to the left hemisphere of the brain, which is the main language centre. Therefore, when the right ear becomes the directing ear, the delay is removed and the stutter can be overcome. Studies with stutterers have indicated the effectiveness of Sound Therapy in between 82 to 100 percent of cases.[64]

Active listening

Listening means that we direct our ears to actively tune in to selected sounds and to tune others out. A person who cannot do this will be unable to follow a conversation in a noisy environment and may therefore appear standoffish or antisocial. Sound Therapy re-educates the selective ability of the ear, enabling listening to become a focused, motivated response to sound.

Sound sensitivity

Sound sensitivity can result from overly acute hearing or from a general state of over-sensitivity in which noise is an irritating stimulant. The ear should naturally possess the ability to modify the intensity of incoming sound. The range and adaptability of the ear is miraculous if you think about the variety of conditions it can handle. It can tolerate noise of quite high decibel levels, like traffic or rock music, and yet, in a quiet environment, it can hear a pin drop. No microphone could possibly have the flexibility and precision of the human ear. When normal sound becomes an irritant, this means that the ear has lost its ability to turn down or tune out unwanted sound. Sound Therapy listeners frequently find that, when the ear is retrained, their noise tolerance improves as the ear regains its full adaptability and responsiveness.

---

63   Tomatis, *The Conscious Ear.* Ibid.
64   Van Jaarsveld, P.E; and Du Plessis, W.F., 'Audio-psycho-phonology at Potchefstroom: a review,' *South Africa Tydskr. Sielk (South African Journal of Psychology)*, Vol.18, No.4, 1988, pp.136-142.

Chronic Fatigue and environmental sensitivity

Chronic Fatigue Syndrome has now been linked to chemical sensitivity.[65] In some cases this broad spectrum acquired sensitivity even extends to electro-magnetic sensitivity, making it hard for a person to tolerate exposure to mobile phones and other electronic devices. While the cause is linked to chemical overload, and removal of the irritants is believed necessary, Sound Therapy can also play a role in recovery. The complexities of the immune system and a body out of balance are just beginning to be unraveled.

The effect of electro-magnetic pollution is even less understood, and it may be in this area that Sound Therapy is of the most significance. Throughout her life Patricia Joudry suffered from sound, chemical and electro-magnetic sensitivity. Sound Therapy was the most significant aid to her in dealing with all of these challenges. Other listeners with chronic fatigue have had similar benefits in terms of energy lifts, better sleep and a greater ability to cope with life. In conjunction with nutritional supplementation and environmental medicine, Sound Therapy can be of benefit for many people with chronic fatigue.

Brain plasticity

Research on brain plasticity in the last few decades has given us a deeper understanding of how Sound Therapy works. At the time when Dr. Tomatis first made his discoveries scientific opinion about the brain was very different from where it stands today. We believed then that the brain had set functions in particular areas which could not change, so if brain damage occurred it was irrevocable. Now science has proven that the brain can form new connections at any stage of life, and that with effort and the right sort of stimulation the brain has a remarkable ability to remap itself and rebuild its

---

65 Crumpler, Diana, *Chemical Crisis*, Scribe Publications, Newham, Australia, 1994. Hilary, E., *Children of a Toxic Harvest*, Lothian, Melbourne, 1997.

functions.[66] It appears therefore, that remapping the brain may be one of the significant positive impacts of Sound Therapy. High frequency, complex fluctuating tones and melodies stimulate both the ear and many areas of the brain involved in music and language. This explains why we can see improvement in so many different areas resulting from Sound Therapy. Building and reorganising our brain pathways can result in better sensory perception, better integration between the senses, better mood, cognition, memory and even co-ordination and physical performance.

The field of brain research is at an exciting point of momentum. Our knowledge of brain plasticity opens a huge horizon of what is possible. Sound Therapy is one of the modalities at the forefront of this research.

Personal stories

The variety of benefits experienced by Sound Therapy listeners seems extraordinary, yet this is only because we fail to recognize the profound importance of the ear to our overall functioning and well-being. The ear is the gateway to the brain. It is linked via the cranial nerves to many other organs and it is the organ by which we orient ourselves in our environment and in relation to others. The stories included in Part Two of this book indicate the remarkable changes that many individuals can experience in life when the function of the ear is improved.

---

66 Doige, N. Ibid.
     Greenfield, Susan, Ibid

Chapter Four

Children, Sound and Learning

> 66 *When we develop listening, we get to the basic, basic skill* 99
> *we've been seeking and talking about for decades. We get to*
> *the problem rather than dealing with the symptoms.*
>
> Billie M. Thompson Ph.D.

Children are fast responders and some of the results they have achieved with Sound Therapy have been remarkable. Larissa, a fourteen-year-old girl who was a talented musician, struggled with learning and social difficulties and sound sensitivity. When she first started to use Sound Therapy she went into her room and listened for a four hour stretch. She came out and the family was all sitting around the table. The girl pointed to a coke bottle on the table and said in astonishment, "Look! I can see the letters! There's space between the letters, I can read it!"

This certainly proves that the senses of sight and hearing are closely interlinked, as an investigation of the pathways of the auditory and oculomotor nerves will confirm. This is why, of course, Dr. Tomatis stressed the importance of auditory re-training to assist children with their reading. "Children read with their ears," he said.

Larissa continued to listen for several weeks, often doing eight or nine hours a day, even keeping it on when she was playing the piano. The results were remarkable in several areas, improving her learning ability, her expressiveness and social skills; and increasing her tolerance for sound.

Sound Therapy is not a panacea for all learning problems but it is a part of the puzzle which, if it is missing, can mean that the whole picture will never come together. The sense of hearing is such an enormous part of the learning process that to endeavour to correct learning without providing some rehabilitation for the ear is almost like attempting to learn to read and write without first learning the alphabet.

Down syndrome

Approximately seventy-five percent of children with Down syndrome have a hearing impairment.[67] This is often due to recurrent middle ear infections and wax impaction. Repeated, chronic middle ear infections result in fibrous adhesions which limit the movement of the three tiny bones in the middle ear, resulting in progressive hearing loss. Down syndrome children also have a higher incidence of sensorineural hearing loss, both congenital and progressive.[68] These children are significantly affected by sensory deprivation and they need preventive measures if they are to reach their full cognitive potential. A delay in the comprehension of language results in a delay in speaking.[69]

The impairment of language abilities delays learning in all areas and makes the task of education and socialisation more difficult. This results in behaviour problems which could be avoided if the language abilities were improved.

Why Sound Therapy helps

It is very important for children with Down syndrome to have their hearing treated in the early years to assist with language development.[70] These children respond well to education in the area of social and emotional adjustment, motor skills and visual comprehension. Their greatest area of difficulty in learning is in auditory vocal processing. They often have difficulty learning to

---

67   Moss, K., 'Hearing and Vision Loss Associated with Down Syndrome,' TSBVI Deafblind Outreach. http://www.deafblind.com/downmoss.html
68   Snashall, S. 'Hearing Impairment and Down's Syndrome.' Cited on 7th Sept 2009: http://www.intellectualdisability.info/complex_disability/P_hearing_ds.htm
69   Rogers, P.T; and Coleman, M., *Medical Care in Down's Syndrome: a Preventive Medicine Approach*, Marcel Dekker, 1992.
70   Madaule, P., 'Down's Syndrome: Becoming Just One of The Kids.' Originally presented at the meeting of the Association for Down's Syndrome of Mexico City in 1989.

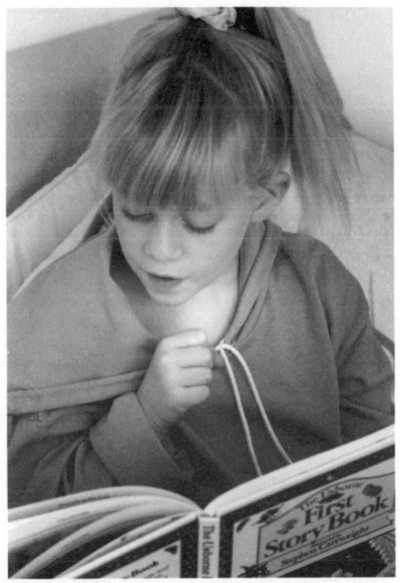

The Reading Aloud exercise

manipulate the speech system, co-ordinating the tongue, lips, jaw and palate. Because they face much greater obstacles in producing speech sounds, they need special assistance with their hearing.

Dr. Tomatis discovered that the voice can only produce what the ear can hear. Sound Therapy stimulates the hearing capacity and exercises the ear, training it in particular to receive high frequency sounds that are lost when hearing is damaged.[71] The sounds of consonants such as b, d, p, g and t, are high frequency sounds that are, of course, essential for clear comprehension of speech and before they can begin learning to produce these sounds, children must first be able to hear them. As Sound Therapy stimulates the brain to enhance perception in the full range of frequencies, a greater range of tonality is made available to the voice. This is very important for the production of intelligible speech.

How to use Sound Therapy with Down syndrome children

Parents should ensure that their children's ears are checked regularly and that they receive treatment for ear infections or wax impaction. In some cases the recurrence of these problems will decrease with the use of Sound Therapy. The movement and exercise produced in the ear by Sound Therapy often results in a spontaneous expulsion of fluid from the ear and blockages may be less likely to recur. It is helpful for children with Down syndrome to listen regularly to Sound Therapy on a long-term, permanent basis, to protect the ear against its tendency to become easily blocked and to stimulate the full range of hearing. [72]

The auditory stimulation provided by Sound Therapy has a recharging effect on the brain, and children with Down syndrome generally respond with enthusiasm. It is important to continue language education throughout the life of a person with Down syndrome and this ongoing learning process will be greatly enhanced by listening to Sound Therapy for people of any age.

---

71   Ibid.
72   Madaule, P., Ibid.

What it achieves

The protection and enhancement of hearing that can be achieved through Sound Therapy has significant results for all areas of development of children with Down syndrome. Improved hearing results in more liveliness and willingness to learn, which leads to a greater interest in the person's environment and daily activities. Language comprehension and speech improve significantly and, because the links between learning language and learning about the world are direct, not only education but performance in all areas will be enhanced.[73]

Dyslexia

Dyslexia, meaning "reading difficulty" was originally called "word blindness" and thought to be a visual problem. One of the earliest writers on the subject, Dr. Hinshelwood, was an eye surgeon, which may account for the initial emphasis on visual difficulties. Many more recent studies point to language and auditory problems as the fundamental cause.[74, 75]

Listening is the most basic skill required for verbal communication and a weakness in listening ability will hinder the development of a strong language base. Consequently, the child encounters problems when the time comes to approach the more complex linguistic tasks of writing and reading. If the sounds of speech have not been accurately heard, they cannot be accurately conveyed by symbols.

The left hemisphere of the brain is the main center for processing language. In order for speech sounds to reach the brain efficiently the right ear must take a leading role in listening, because the right ear communicates most directly with the left brain hemisphere.

---

73 Ibid.
74 Dougherty, R.F; et al., 'Dichotic pitch: a new stimulus distinguishes normal and dyslexic auditory function,' *Neuro Report,* Vol. 9, No.13, Auditory and Vestibular Systems, 14 September 1998, pp.3001-3005.
75 Hari, R. and Kiesilä, P., 'Deficit of temporal auditory processing in dyslexic adults,' Low Temperature Laboratory, Helsinki University of Technology, 02150, Espoo, Finland, March 1999.

Dr. Tomatis argued that children with dyslexia have failed to achieve right ear dominance and that therefore the order in which they hear sound becomes jumbled. If they sometimes use the left and sometimes the right ear as the directing ear, sounds may reach the brain at different speeds, so letters will be jumbled. This accounts for errors of reversal, such as writing "was" as "saw" or pronouncing "spaghetti" as "pisghetti."

Why Sound Therapy helps

The balance between the two hemispheres of the brain is of fundamental importance in overcoming dyslexia. Both hemispheres play a role in processing language, but the roles they play are different. The eye must combine with the power and the quality of the ear to make sense of the written sounds. This co-ordination happens easily when the left hemisphere deals primarily with audition and the right hemisphere deals primarily with vision. In dyslexia, the route which allows for phonic analysis has been damaged. Several studies have supported Tomatis's discovery that Sound Therapy can restore the functioning of this route and reduce or eliminate the cause of the problem.[76]

Tomatis says "We read with our ears ... the ear is the organ of language, the pathway to language assimilation, the key that controls it, the receptor regulating its flow."[77]

Sound Therapy, according to Tomatis and his proponents, stimulates and exercises the ear, teaching it to receive and interpret sound in an efficient manner.[78] Music is a highly organised series of sounds that the ear has to analyse. Therefore, listening to music is an excellent way for a child to learn how to perceive sounds in an organised fashion, or in other words, to listen. The higher volume of sound to the right ear, which is built into all Sound Therapy recordings, means that the right ear is educated to be the directing ear. When

---

76 Gilmor, T.M. 'The Efficacy of the Tomatis Method for Children with Learning and Communication disorders; A Meta Analysis,' Ibid, pp.12-23.
77 Tomatis, A.A., *The Conscious Ear*, Ibid.
78 Weeks, Ibid, See Appendix 2.

this right ear dominance is achieved, the problem of reversal will frequently disappear.

What it achieves

Children with dyslexia often have feelings of inferiority after repeated failure. It is unfair that they must try many times harder than anyone else to achieve only mediocre results. Sound Therapy can offer immediate emotional relief because it is a method of treatment that does not require any extra effort from the child. As there is no need to struggle with the problem area of language, the child is let off the hook for once and is able to enjoy a treatment that is not a constant reminder of his or her apparent inadequacies.[79]

Once the basic cause of the language difficulties is remedied by Sound Therapy, and the child is able to receive and interpret sound accurately and easily, his or her ability and motivation to communicate is greatly increased. Thus the problem learner is transformed into a receptive and motivated learner.[80]

The reading aloud exercise

Children who are experiencing difficulty with reading should begin the reading aloud exercise after they have completed ten to twenty hours of listening. The child sits in an erect but comfortable posture and reads aloud while holding the right hand near the mouth, as though holding an imaginary microphone. This has the psychological effect of "switching on" the voice. At the same time it encourages right ear dominance, which is necessary for the successful conversion of visual symbols into sound. This exercise should be done for fifteen minutes each day, and can be continued until the reading problems are resolved.

---

79 Madaule, Paul, 'The Dyslexified World', in *About the Tomatis Method*, edited by Gilmor, T. M; Madaule, P; and Thompson, B., The Listening Centre Press, Toronto, 1989.

80 Madaule, Paul, *When Listening comes Alive. A Guide to Effective Learning and Communication*, Ibid.
Joudry, R. *Why Aren't I Learning?* Sound Therapy International, Sydney, 2004.

Pre-natal listening

Sound is the first sense to develop fully in the womb. The foetus's ear is ready to perceive sound at four-and-a-half months. The baby listens to its mother's heartbeat, respiration and digestive sounds. Dr.Tomatis believed that the baby can also hear the mother's voice and becomes familiar with this sound before birth. Tomatis discovered that all of the sound heard in utero is high frequency (above 8,000 Hz) due to the development of the embryonic ear. Birth is an often traumatic event in which the child is pushed from the familiar and protected environment of the womb into a totally unknown world, to begin the process of learning to communicate with others.

The effect of Sound Therapy

The sound of the mother's voice with its familiar tone and rhythm is what provides continuity between the prenatal and post-natal worlds. The infant is particularly accustomed to the high frequency sounds of the voice as heard in the womb, and therefore is immediately reassured when presented with high frequency sounds filtered to a similar level.

When the mother listens to Sound Therapy during her pregnancy, the benefits she receives are passed on to the infant. The effects of listening for the mother are a soothing of her whole system and a stimulation to the cortex of the brain from the high frequency sound.[81] Because of its connection with the vital vagus nerve (the tenth cranial nerve) the ear plays a part in nearly everything we feel, including heartbeat and breathing or sensations like a tickle in the throat or butterflies in the stomach.[82] The positive effects of the Sound Therapy are therefore passed through the mother's whole body and have an influence on the development of the foetus.

---

81 Whitwell, G. E., 'The Importance of Prenatal Sound and Music,' *The Journal of Prenatal and Perinatal Psychology and Health.*
82 Weeks, Bradford, S., 'The Therapeutic Effect of High Frequency Audition and its Role in Sacred Music,' See Appendix 2.

The hormonal shift experienced by the mother at birth sometimes causes post-natal depression. This can be greatly alleviated by the continued use of Sound Therapy after giving birth, as well as by herbal treatment to balance the hormones, such as the topical application of wild yam cream.[83]

Effects for the infant

We have heard of a child born to a mother who had been listening regularly to Sound Therapy. Straight after birth the headphones were placed on the baby's ears and it immediately stopped crying, perhaps feeling relieved of the sudden isolation and separateness.[84] Babies born of mothers who listened to Sound Therapy during pregnancy show a distinct lack of tension and anxiety as they grow.[85] They have an inner peacefulness and are less reactive, making them easier to manage. They feel secure in their relationship with their mother and will go easily to other people. They also have a natural appreciation for classical music and can continue to benefit from its healing properties. It is also beneficial for these children to listen to Sound Therapy as they grow, in order to facilitate their development of communication and language skills.

Autism

Autism is a brain development disorder which causes children to become emotionally isolated from the world around them. It is often characterised by restricted and repetitive behavior. Some decades ago autism was attributed to a lack of affection in the child's mother. Though Dr. Tomatis, being a product of his time, believed in this view, it is no longer considered valid.

Due to a greater research emphasis on genetic factors in recent years, many scientists believe there may be a genetic cause to autism, but more evidence is now pointing to environmental causes such as mercury and other heavy metals, pesticides and chemicals in the

83 Shealy, C. N., Ibid.
84 Private conversation with Patricia Joudry.
85 Private conversation with Francoise Nicolof.

home such as flame retardants. Many new household items such as mattresses, carpets, cars and furniture are treated with flame retardants which give off harmful chemical gases which enter the body via the respiratory system.[86]

A question has been raised by a number of parents' groups about a possible link between autism and vaccines, and it is important that this area should be fully researched. At Swinburne University in Melbourne, a 20-year study found favourable comparisons with homoeopathic 'vaccination.' Evidence suggests that homoeoprophylaxis (homoeopathic 'vaccination') is a valid alternative method and may in fact assist the maturation of the immune system.[87]

Children with developmental disorders often suffer from food sensitivities and digestive problems, making it harder for them to rid the body of toxins. They also have an imbalance of seratonin and tryptophan, brain chemicals important for affecting mood and emotion. These conditions form part of a syndrome of environmentally-related health problems. Research has shown that treatment with pro-biotics (healthy gut flora) can make a significant difference, helping to improve detoxification and balance brain chemistry.[88]

Environmental medicine is exploring this area. However this field has received only limited recognition and funding, as it poses a major paradigm shift away from the pre-eminence of pharmaceutical

---

86 Madsen, Lee, and Olle, 'Growing Threats: Toxic Flame Retardants and Children's Health,' Environment California Research and Policy Center, Mar, 2003. Cited on 24th Aug 09, http://www.mindfully.org/Plastic/Flame/Children-Flame-RetardantsMar03.htm

87 Golden, I., 'Homoeoprophylaxis – a Proven Alternative to Vaccination,' *Nourished Magazine*, Dec, 2008.

88 Wakefield AJ, et al, 'Ileal-lymphoid-nodular hyperplasia, non-specific colitis, and pervasive developmental disorder in children,' *Lancet,* 351 (9103) Feb 28 1998, pp.637-41.
Parracho, H. et al. 'Differences between the gut microflora of children with autistic spectrum disorders and that of healthy children,' *J Med Microbiol*, 54, 2005, pp.987-991.
Hoshino, Y. et al., 'Blood Serotonin and Free Tryptophan Concentration in Autistic Children,' *Neuropsychobiology,* Vol.11, 1984, pp.22-27.

solutions. The increasing incidence of autism in recent decades certainly points to environmental toxins as the cause.

Autism rates have increased significantly in recent years, from one in 500 ten years ago, up to one in 150 children born today. It has become the fastest growing developmental disability and is increasing at 10 to 17% per year.[89]

Without pinpointing the cause, there is widespread agreement that one of the factors in autism is a distortion in the reception of sensory information. Many children with autism exhibit extreme sensitivity to noise. Some frequencies are actually painful for them to hear.

Dr. Tomatis suggested that in order to shut out painful sounds or other unwanted stimuli the child closes down the hearing mechanism so that certain sounds cannot penetrate the consciousness. On a physiological level, this closing off of the ear is achieved by a relaxation of the muscles of the middle ear. Over time, these muscles lose their tonicity, and the brain pathways intended for auditory reception do not develop properly. Sounds are then imprecisely perceived and as a result incorrectly analysed.

Sensory integration is a fascinating field which examines the ability of the conscious mind to integrate information from the various senses such as hearing and sight and touch. Anomalies or differences in this process mean that some people with autism may be highly literate, and able to write, yet unable to look you in the eye or have even the most basic conversation.

Although they may understand what is said to them, they are unable to process and have tuned out many of the frequencies in the sound, and have thus tuned out the emotional content of the message.

---

89 'Investigating the Environmental Origins of Autism,' July 8, 2008, see: http://www.scientificamerican.com/article.cfm?id=investigating-environmental-origins-of-autism

Why Sound Therapy helps

Sound Therapy offers a child with autism the opportunity to re-open the listening capacity. The fluctuating sounds produced by the Electronic Ear provide stimulation which, according to Tomatis's theory, will gradually exercise and tone the ear muscles, teaching the ear to respond to and recognise the full range of frequencies. This in turn assists with building integration in the brain between sounds and other sensory inputs. As this happens, communication takes on new meanings and the child begins to respond, where before he or she was unreachable.[90]

Tomatis explains that Sound Therapy recreates the pre-birth experience of audition and enables emotional contact to be made first with the mother and then with other people.[91]

There have been some fascinating books about individual experiences of recovery from autism using a type of sound therapy. One was *The Sound of a Miracle* by Annabel Stehli, about her daughter Georgie's significant recovery from autism using Dr. Berard's adaptation of the Tomatis method in the 1980s.[92]

The other, *Lucy's Story* by Lucy Blackman, is by a young woman who, though unable to develop any verbal communication skills, was able with the help of assisted communication and Sound Therapy to write her own story. Her lucid description of how she experienced the world and how sound therapy helped to integrate her senses is very enlightening.[93]

She writes: "the most wonderful thing had happened, though. I could not speak myself, but for the first time I now could understand what speech was. ... The phenomenon of speech as a human attribute

---

90 Gilmor, T. 'The Efficacy of the Tomatis Method for Children with Learning and Communication disorders; A Meta Analysis,' Ibid, pp.12-23.
91 Tomatis, A.A., *The Conscious Ear*, Ibid.
92 Stehli, A., *The Sound of a Miracle: A Child's Triumph over Autism*, New York, Doubleday, 1991.
93 Blackman, L., *Lucy's Story: Autism and Other Adventures*, Book In Hand, Brisbane, 1999.

suddenly became explicable, in the way that swimming may make the phenomenon of gravity explicable."

There have also been many, many accounts of improvement in children on the autism spectrum using the Tomatis method and the portable, Joudry, adaptation.[94], [95]

How to use Sound Therapy with autism

Many children with autism instinctively love the Sound Therapy program and will listen to it readily, even being willing to wear headphones which they might otherwise reject. In other cases ingenuity may be needed to get the child to wear headphones, but it is well worth the effort. The self-help method has the advantage of enabling regular, long-term listening over a period of several months. For children with autism a long-term treatment program may be necessary.

To support the changes being introduced by Sound Therapy it may be important to also introduce dietary changes and nutritional supplements. Because toxic accumulation and digestive problems are common in children with autism, this multi-pronged approach can be very important. Discuss your choice of pro-biotics with your Sound Therapy consultant to ensure you find an effective one.

What it achieves

Sound Therapy has the potential to make a child's perception of sound more accurate and normal,[96] so that they can begin to experience the world and other people the way the rest of us do. Children with autism generally respond to Sound Therapy by showing a greater interest in making contact and communicating with the people around them. Interactions with their family members become more affectionate and appropriate. There is often increased eye contact and the children have a longer attention span. They will initiate

---

94 Gilmor, T. M. and Madaule, P. 'Opening Communication: a New Perspective on Autism,' in *About the Tomatis Method*, edited by Gilmor, T. M., Madaule, P. and Thompson, B., The Listening Centre Press, Toronto, 1989.
95 Joudry, R., Ibid.
96 Tomatis, A. A. *The Ear and Language*, Ibid.

contact rather than waiting to be approached. For children without language, vocalisation often increases, initially as screams and then as babbling. Children who can speak develop a more appropriate use of language, for instance, beginning to use more personal pronouns ("I", "you") or first names, and using words to express their feelings. They begin to laugh and cry at appropriate times. Once children begin to emerge from their emotional isolation they will show increasing responsiveness to what they are being taught, and to the people who care for them.[97]

Attention Deficit Disorder

Attention Deficit Disorder (ADD) and Attention Deficit and Hyperactivity Disorder (ADHD) are names given to a collection of symptoms that have become common in the last 20 to 30 years. These include an inability to focus the attention, being easily distractible, restless and hyperactive. An official diagnosis simply means that a doctor has given the child a high enough score on a rating scale of these symptoms, based on observations at a clinic visit. A child who displays similar symptoms but does not receive the diagnosis is simply at a lower point on the scale, as the diagnosis is really a fairly arbitrary decision based on the judgment of the clinician at the time of the visit.

Attention deficit hyperactivity disorder (ADHD) affects somewhere between 10% and 15% of all school children in the U.S. (1.8 million to 2.7 million children), and is on the increase. At first considered a psychological problem and then a congenital brain disorder, emerging evidence now says ADHD is mainly caused by chemical and environmental factors.[98] The significant increase in neuro-developmental disorders over the past 30 years can only be explained by our increasing exposure to environmental contaminants.

---

97 Gilmor, T. M. and Madaule, P., Ibid.
    Joudry, R. Ibid.
98 Luke T. C, and Kalpana P., 'Nutritional and Environmental Approaches to Preventing and Treating Autism and Attention Deficit Hyperactivity Disorder (ADHD): A Review,' *The Journal of Alternative and Complementary Medicine*, 14(1) January/February 2008, pp.79-85.

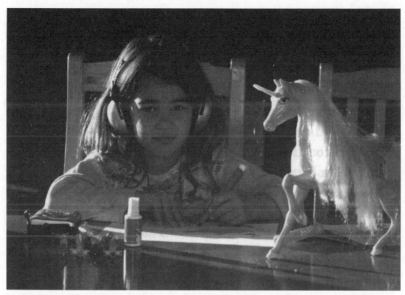

Talina loves to listen while she is painting and drawing

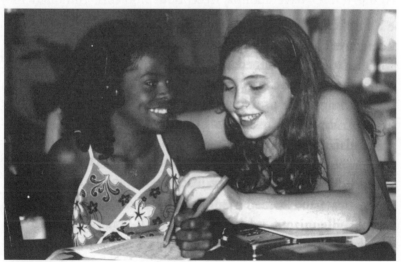

Sound Therapy helps children to be relaxed and focussed when doing their homework

Food dyes, preservatives and artificial sweeteners along with heavy metals and other agricultural and industrial chemicals, all combine to upset the delicate balance of neurotransmitters in the brain.

The impact of environmental toxins on children's health has become a major concern to the US government, resulting in a focus on research by the EPA and the National Institute of Environmental Health Sciences (NIEHS).[99] Philippe Grandjean, adjunct professor at Harvard School of Public Health said "The brains of our children are our most precious economic resource, and we haven't recognized how vulnerable they are." As the lead author of a study published in *The Lancet* , he stated, "We must make protection of the young brain a paramount goal of public health protection. You have only one chance to develop a brain." [100]

The symptoms of ADD/ADHD are believed to be caused by a deficiency in the transmission system which relays messages between cells in various parts of the brain. The majority of children with ADD/ADHD have auditory reception problems. Although they can hear, they cannot make sense of what they hear, because the ear and the brain are not working efficiently to process the sound. They have difficulty tuning out unwanted input and focusing on selected sounds.

This indiscriminate reception of auditory input is linked to the inability to concentrate on a selected topic for any length of time. Where hyperactivity is part of the child's condition, there are additional problems of impulsiveness, behavioural problems and poor social skills.

99   Gupta, M.S., 'Neurodevelopmental Disorders in Children - Autism and ADHD.' EnvironmentalChemistry.com. April 14 2008. Accessed on-line: 8/26/2009 http://EnvironmentalChemistry.com/yogi/environmental/200804childrenautismadhd.html

100 Grandjean, P; Landrigan, P., 'Developmental neurotoxicity of industrial chemicals,' *The Lancet*, Vol. 368, No. 9553, pp.2167-2178.

Why Sound Therapy helps ADD/ADHD

Tomatis has suggested that Sound Therapy retrains the listening capacity (or the auditory reception process) so that the child can learn to focus on the desired sound and to relay the sound directly to the language centre in the brain.[101] The full stimulation provided to the sensory systems is believed to repair damaged brain pathways and improve the production and uptake of important neurotransmitters.[102, 103]

Tomatis theorized that when auditory reception problems occur, the child uses longer, less efficient brain pathways. Studies have found that by stimulating the auditory pathways with Sound Therapy to improve audio-vocal conditioning, brain function and control of attention improve.[104] This process reduces stress and tension in the whole nervous system as the child becomes able to attend to a chosen stimulus, instead of being constantly distracted by every sound in the environment.

What it achieves

Noticeable improvements may occur quickly with Sound Therapy for children with ADD/ADHD. Parents and teachers commonly report improvement in both behaviour and academic performance. One change that is often observed is a marked decrease in activity (for overactive children) while underactive children may become more energized. As the listening discrimination is retrained, memory and concentration improve, so that learning can be achieved with a great deal less effort. Sleep and appetite problems are resolved as the whole system becomes calmer and less erratic. The behavioural difficulties, such as impulsiveness and aggression, are now brought down to a manageable level. The child is now able to pay attention

---

101 Tomatis, A. A. *The Ear and Language*, Ibid.
102 Sekulowicz, M.G., 'The Role Of Early Diagnosis And Therapy Of ADHD,' Proceedings of the Tenth Biennial Conference of the International Association of Special Education, Hong Kong, June 2007.
103 *The Mindd Handbook: An Integrative approach to treating ADHD, Allergies, Autism, Asthma and Neuro-biological illness*, The MINDD Foundation, 2007. www.mindd.org
104 Gilmor, T, 'The Efficacy of the Tomatis Method for Children with Learning and Communication disorders; A Meta Analysis,' Ibid, pp.12-23.

in class and to understand and follow instructions; and is motivated to communicate and learn.

A study by Davis in Rockaway New Jersey in 2005 evaluated the impact of 60 hours of Tomatis training on 11 ADD/ADHD children. The following table shows the percentage of children who improved on a variety of aptitudes, according to observations by parents.[105]

Davis study: percentage of ADD/ADHD children who improved according to parents' observations.	
Ability or Behaviour	%
Interpersonal growth	82
Listening and speech	91
Academic achievement	91
Attention	100
Behaviour	91
Personal growth	82
Movement, sports, rhythm	64
Musical and vocal skills	55
Relaxation	73
Creativity	64
Reading, writing, spelling	55
Well-being	36

Speech problems

Tomatis has argued that speech is controlled by the ear. According to this theory, unless there is a deformity in the vocal apparatus, most speech difficulties are caused by some interference or distortion in auditory reception.[106] Although the hearing may test

---

105 Gerristen, J., 'A Review of Research done on Tomatis Auditory Stimulation,' http://www.tomatis.com/English/Articles/research.htm
106 Tomatis, A. A., The Ear and Language, Ibid.

as normal, the relaying of verbal information to the brain may be impaired. Confusion in the sequence of received sounds can cause confusion in speech output. Hearing your own voice as a source of constant feedback while speaking, as when you have a poor phone connection with an echo, is a good example of this. The results can be substitutions of one sound for another, stumbling over words or a flat and toneless voice.[107]

Most people use the left hemisphere of the brain as the primary integrating centre for language. Some studies have shown that there are changes in the balance between the right and left hemispheres and how they are used for speech in stutterers.[108] Tomatis said that the right hemisphere is less efficient for processing auditory information, so when it is used as the primary language centre, the result is problems in the timing of speech output.[109]

Speech difficulties frequently lead to problems in other areas where language is used, such as reading and writing. The element which is the basis for all these skills is the ability to hear and process sound accurately.

Why Sound Therapy helps speech problems

Dr. Tomatis made an important discovery about the relatedness of the ear to the voice. He established that the larynx emits only those harmonics that the ear hears. A lack of tone in the voice indicates a lack of tone in the hearing. Sound Therapy fine tunes the hearing and restores the ability to perceive frequencies essential for speech by stimulating the ear and the brain pathways in the auditory cortex.[110] It also corrects reversed or mixed laterality, so that the left hemisphere performs efficiently as the processing centre for language.[111] This is achieved by continually playing more sound

---

107 Ibid.
108 Salmelin, R.; Schnitzler, A.; Schmitz, F.; Jäncke, L.; Witte, O.W.; Freund, H.-J., 'Functional organization of the auditory cortex is different in stutterers and fluent speakers,' NeuroReport, Vol. 9, No.10, 13 July 1998, pp.2225-2229.
109 Tomatis, A. A., The Ear and Language, Ibid.
110 Ibid.
111 Ibid.

into the right ear. The right ear connects to the left hemisphere of the brain, so when the right ear becomes dominant, the language function naturally switches to the left hemisphere.[112]

Listening for speech

Regular daily listening is essential for the right ear dominance to be achieved.[113] The *Let's Recite* album is good to use for children with speech difficulties as it gives them the opportunity to repeat back what is said and integrate their speaking with their new experience of listening. Another good exercise for children with any form of speech difficulty is speaking into a microphone while monitoring their voice through the right ear. This can be done using a recording Walkman with a microphone and wearing only the right headphone. The child can speak, sing, read or make any vocal sounds. A similar effect can be achieved without the equipment by simply closing off the right ear with fingers or an ear plug. This increases the volume of the child's own voice in the right ear. This exercise can be done for some time each day in conjunction with the listening.

What it achieves

Dr. Tomatis and other practitioners using his method have had considerable success with stutterers by educating them to be right ear dominant.[114] We have seen the same results for those listening to our portable Sound Therapy. Children with other types of speech difficulties have responded similarly to the treatment. Not only does their speech improve but their behaviour changes. They become more confident, more dynamic and more eager to talk and communicate. Parents also report on improvements in reading and the use of written language.

---

112 Ibid.
113 Tomatis, A.A., *The Conscious Ear*, Ibid.
114 Van Jaarsveld, P.E. and du Plessis, W.F., Ibid.

How to organise your child's listening program

Regular listening to Sound Therapy is essential to achieve successful results. The child should listen every day, if possible for between 30 and 60 minutes. If the child wishes to listen for longer than this each day, that will be even more beneficial. Develop a listening routine that suits your child.

Listening can be done during sleep, play, homework or travel. If the child wishes to listen at school, parents can ask for the consent of the teacher. This will likely be granted, as listening in the classroom will often help the child to concentrate and perform better.

Sound Therapy should never be forced on a child, as this would cause resistance and be counter productive to the aim of opening the listening capacity. It should be presented as an enjoyable activity and the benefits should be explained in a way that is appropriate for the child. This gives an opportunity to teach children to value their hearing. They can learn about how the ears work and the importance of not damaging them. There is nothing wrong with offering incentives to persuade the child to listen. The promise of a reward once the child has done, say, 100 hours of listening, may prove effective in some cases.

Children rarely object to wearing headphones unless for some reason they are uncomfortable. It is a good idea to have two different types of headphones in case one becomes uncomfortable for the child. If your child is too hyperactive to wear the headphones you can put them on at night while the child is sleeping. The mini phones which sit inside the outer ear can be taped in with surgical tape to stop them from falling out during sleep. Be sure to place the headphone marked R in the right ear. For listening during sleep the music albums are most suitable.

The volume should never be too loud, as any loud sound damages the ear. It should be just loud enough for the child to hear comfortably. If the child is listening while going to sleep, the volume can be turned down very low.

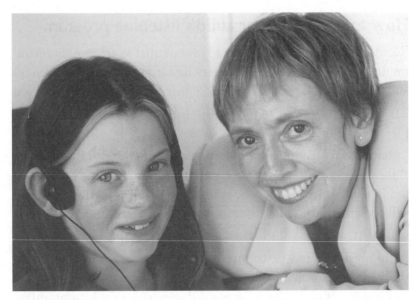

Rafaele Joudry with Emily, who makes friends more easily since using Sound Therapy

The total listening time required for most children to receive a noticeable benefit from the program is approximately 100 hours. Although some children will begin to achieve results in the first few days of listening, they should still continue listening as the longer they listen, the more advantages they will gain. Just like physical exercise, Sound Therapy supports a child's healthy development through life.

Most children have an instinctive response to the acoustic stimulation of Sound Therapy and will take to the listening keenly.

Long-term listening and other treatment
For children with mild to moderate conditions

Once the child has completed 100 hours of listening, which may take two to four months of daily routine, the hours can be reduced if desired. It is beneficial to still listen on a regular basis or as often as the child wants to, as this will help to maintain the positive results.

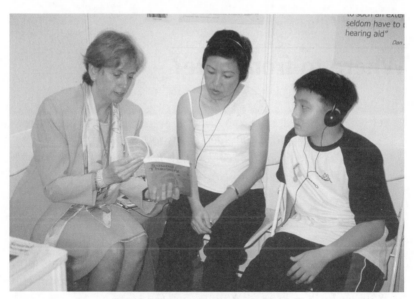

Sound Therapy is an aid to study and concentration

For children with profound conditions

It should be noted that for treating children with profound conditions, such as autism or severe dyslexia, a long-term listening program may be beneficial. Retraining new aptitudes in the brain can take many months and even years.[115] In these cases, several hundred hours of listening may be required to see significant benefits. To conduct an effective listening program parents will need to make a long-term commitment to supervising their child's listening. It is vitally important to give the child regular Sound Therapy as early as possible, as pathways in the lower levels of the brain become less adaptable as the child matures.[116] The child will also benefit from other forms of treatment, such as counselling, speech therapy or remedial reading lessons, and these will complement the effects of Sound Therapy.

115 Doige, N., Ibid.
116 Harrison, R.V., 'Representing the Acoustic World within the Brain: Normal and Abnormal Development of Frequency Maps in the Auditory System,' Conference Keynote Address. Proceedings of the 2nd International Conference, Sponsored by Phonak.

Chapter Five

Where to from here?

Two roads diverged in a wood, and I,
I took the one less travelled by,
And that has made all the difference.

Robert Frost

Now that you have followed the story of Sound Therapy from Tomatis to the present, you may be left with a number of questions. Can it really be as good as it sounds? Will my doctor recommend it? Will my husband use it? Will it work for me?

We can't know exactly how it will work for you because your nervous system is unique and each person responds in a slightly different way. What we do know is that the brain responds to stimulus; the more stimulation you receive the more your brain becomes connected, empowered and revitalized.[117] And, as Philippe Grandjean has pointed out, you only have one chance to develop a brain. But the great discovery of the last 20 years is that this chance is re-presented to us every day of our lives. As Norman Doige, author of the best selling book *The Brain That Changes Itself* likes to remind us, we have the choice to "use it or lose it."[118] It's great to stimulate the brain with conversation, physical exercise, crosswords, learning languages, singing or playing a musical instrument. And all of these, plus anything else we do, may be enhanced and magnified if matched with regular Sound Therapy listening, because stimulation with one sense can increase the function of another.[119]

---

117 Harrison, R.V., Ibid.
118 Doige, N., Ibid.
119 Anastasio, T. J., and Patton, P. E., 'A Two-Stage Unsupervised Learning Algorithm Reproduces Multisensory Enhancement in a Neural Network Model of the Corticotectal System,' *The Journal of Neuroscience*, 23(17) July 30, 2003, pp.6713-6727.

When it comes to the ear, it is so important to ensure that you receive beneficial sound to keep the brain pathways active and alive, and the Sound Therapy program is specifically tailored to enhance and protect our ear function through life. Sadly, it is only when the ears begin to fail that many of us realize how precious they were. I feel blessed that, through my mother's difficulties, I came across this treatment early and have used it for 30 years in the prime of my life, giving me a greater chance than most of retaining good hearing into old age. Choosing to make Sound Therapy part of your life is a positive step for enhancing well-being and choosing to dance the melody, sing the song, and squeeze all the goodness out of life that you possibly can. It's easy to do, fits effortlessly into the busiest schedule, and may help you to reach your potential in an area that you hadn't expected.

I have shared what I know about the results people are seeing and about the science as we understand it today. The rest is up to you.

Sound Therapy product information on last page.

Sound Therapy Self Assessment

This questionnaire will identify areas where your ear/brain functioning may show some weakness and could potentially benefit from Sound Therapy.

		Circle letter if answer is yes or sometimes
		A B C D E
1	Do you often have to ask people to repeat themselves?	A
2	Are you surrounded by machine noise [factory, computer, photocopier, traffic etc] for a large part of each day?	B
3	Do you live in a quiet place with no or very little machine noise?	C
4	Did you have a lot of ear infections as a child?	D
5	Are you troubled by tinnitus (noise in the ears – ringing, buzzing, hissing etc) either continuously or at frequent intervals?	E
6	Do you often have trouble sleeping?	B
7	Do you sleep well and normally wake refreshed?	C
8	Do you have trouble following the ideas when you read?	D
9	Have you had ear or sinus infections which left you with ringing in the ears?	E
10	Does your family complain that you are deaf?	A
11	Do you often long for peace and quiet?	B
12	Are you usually energetic and active?	C
13	Does your tinnitus bother you frequently?	E
14	Have you had tinnitus for a long time?	E
15	Do you have trouble following a conversation in a noisy room?	A
16	Do you use a hearing aid?	A
17	Are you usually exhausted at the end of the day?	B
18	Do you like language and communicate easily?	C
19	Do you have trouble expressing yourself in words or following instructions?	D
20	Do your ears often feel blocked?	E
21	Are you extremely sensitive to noise and have to stay away from it?	A

		A	B	C	D	E
22	Do you like loud music and enjoy going to loud concerts?		B			
23	Do you have difficulty pronouncing complicated words?				D	
24	Does your tinnitus cause you to feel anxious or depressed?					E
25	Have you always had trouble being able to sing in tune?	A				
26	Do your ears ring for some time after being exposed to loud noise?					E
27	Have you always been a poor speller?				D	
28	Are you troubled by dizziness or vertigo or loss of balance?					E
29	Does your hearing affect your social life?	A				
30	Do you have poor memory and concentration?				D	
31	Do you suffer from lack of energy?		B			
32	Do you need more hours of sleep than you would like to?		B			
33	Do you have difficulty making sense of what people are saying?				D	
34	Do you find you have problems learning new languages?				D	
Add up circled letters and write total of each letter in box at bottom of column						
		A	B	C	D	E

Your answers to the questions above will indicate how you may have been affected by noise. Whether you have a high score or a low score, the purpose of this questionnaire is to identify in which areas Sound Therapy is most likely to help you. Was your highest score A's, B's C's D's or E's?

To find our what this means, speak to the practitioner who gave you this book, or call Sound Therapy International (contact details on last page) and speak to one of our qualified health consultants, or complete the assessment online at: www.SoundTherapyInternational. com./self_assessment.htm

(children's assessment also available.)

When you contact us with your results, to thank you for completing this Self Assessment we will be happy to send you a free information pack on Sound Therapy with a DVD and a free gift.

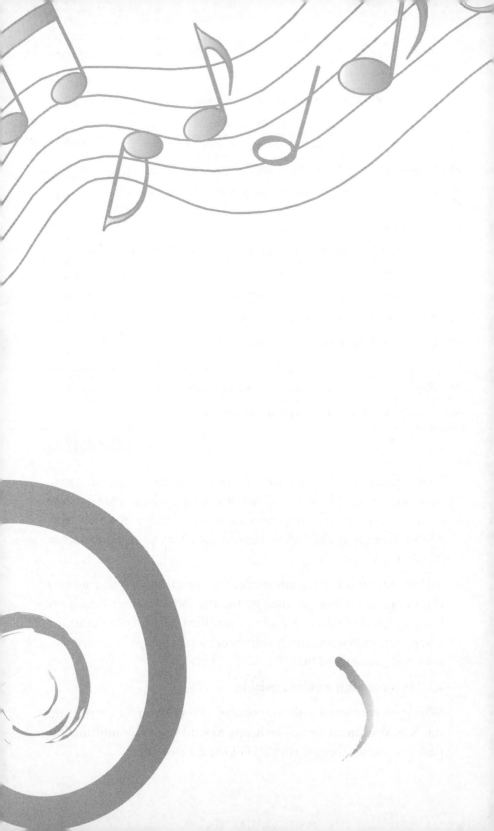

Questions and Answers

Commonly asked questions and answers about Sound Therapy

Q. What equipment do I need to buy to play Sound Therapy?

A. Sound Therapy must be played through headphones to gain the therapeutic effect, and a high quality portable music player engineered to specifications required for Sound Therapy is essential. As technology frequently changes, speak to your Sound Therapy Consultant or visit the website where you ordered this book for information on current recommendations.

Q. Can I play Sound Therapy through speakers?

A. You need to use headphones in order to get the true benefit of the therapy. If you wish to use your home stereo with headphones that is fine, but it will not allow you the mobility of the portable player so it may be hard for you to put in the required listening hours. When using Sound Therapy for a baby that is too young to wear headphones, an alternative is to set up speakers on the right and left of the crib so that the baby will get the correct right left balance.

Q. Why can't I hear any sound in the left ear?

A. You will hear the sound in the left ear if you remove the right headphone and listen to the left one alone. The sound is intentionally louder in the right ear as this stimulates the brain to process sound more efficiently.

Q. What is the tssst-tssst sound in the music?

A. That sound is the therapy! It is caused by the Electronic Ear boosting the high frequencies and that is the sound that stimulates the ear and brain.

Q. How can I find the time to listen?

A. It takes no time at all to listen to Sound Therapy because you can listen on the run, literally. With your personal music player you can listen while you are jogging, reading, sleeping, studying, watching TV, travelling to work, working on the computer, having a conversation or almost any other activity.

Q. Why is the Sound Therapy music so expensive?

A. In fact the Joudry self-help Sound Therapy program is the least expensive way to use Sound Therapy. As compared to over $20.00 per hour for clinical treatment, this program works out at less than $2.00 per hour! Also because you purchase the program yourself you are able to use it for as long a period as required to obtain maximum benefit. For some conditions, listening for several months may be required, and there is no additional cost to you. You can also share the program with other members of your family. Sound Therapy albums are recorded using the highest quality mastering and filtering system, to ensure that you will receive the full therapeutic benefit by playing the original albums. Do not attempt to copy or download the music onto a different playback system or you will lose much of its therapeutic effect. However, if an album ever becomes damaged in any way, we guarantee to replace it for a minimal replacement cost. Remember that when you purchase the Sound Therapy program you are purchasing a highly specialized therapy course, which is completely different to purchasing ordinary music for listening pleasure. You will also receive our ongoing support and advice to help you obtain the maximum benefit from your listening program.

Q. Why is this program so much cheaper than the clinical Tomatis treatment?

A. Because this is a self-help program. Patricia Joudry and the Benedictine monks of Saskatchewan believed that Sound Therapy should be made available to as many people as possible at an affordable cost. Therefore you do not need to pay for a practitioner's time or the use of their facilities. There is no testing required and it is up to you to conduct your own program. As long as you have read one of the Joudry Sound Therapy books and the Self-help Workbook that comes with the kit, you have enough information to conduct your listening program successfully.

Q. Are there additional albums to use after the Basic Kit?

A. Yes, we have a range of several advanced level kits for those who require more variety or who want to take their listening to a higher level. Information on the additional kits will be sent to you with your Basic Kit.

Q. Should I make a copy of the albums and use the copy to preserve the original?

A. No. Each album is made on specialized equipment, required to accurately reproduce the special filtering effects, and if you make copies on other equipment you will lose much of the therapeutic effect of the program. You would be wasting your time listening to an inferior album. There is no problem with using the originals because if one of your albums gets damaged we will replace it for a minimal replacement fee.

Appendix

Excerpts on Tomatis from: 'The Therapeutic effect of high-frequency audition'

The full text of this article is available on: http://weeksmd. com/?p=714

© Dr. Bradford S. Weeks M.D. 1986

Reprinted with kind permission.

> *Every sickness is a musical problem. The healing, therefore, is a musical resolution. The shorter the resolution, the greater is the musical talent of the doctor.*

Abstract:

> *He that hath ears to hear, let him hear.*
>
> Matthew 11:15

This report presents a reinterpretation of the currently accepted theories of human audition. The anatomic structure and the neuro-physiologic functions of the human ear are re-examined. A discussion of the theoretical underpinnings of an intriguing form of sound therapy, filtered high-frequency audition, is presented. The therapy itself is described as well as the patient population, which has benefited from this innovative approach over the past two decades.

Introduction:

In all matters of opinion, our adversaries are deranged

Twain

Through evaluating the controversies which rage within the field of neuro-audiology, it became quite clear that, in times of intellectual upheaval when one theory is attacked by another, qualities of courage and fidelity to scientific methodology are absolutely essential. Courage may be derived from a love of truth. Fidelity involves the ceaseless effort to concentrate, without bias or preconceptions, on the phenomenon itself. To perceive an object, without being waylaid into perception of one's concept thereof, is a profoundly challenging task. It is the keystone of a sound scientific edifice.

Therefore, when presented with interpretations which seemed far-fetched, it was an exercise in tolerance to reserve judgement until the case had been made in its entirety. An attitude of "reserve and observe" had to be cultivated. Only then, I found, can the data be appreciated from a new and exciting light. Children of convenience, we are often placated by the original interpretation of data and there it may sit atop its laurels, an incumbent theory, defying reinterpretation despite the advance of technology. In time, most theories yield to reformulation due to their inherent weaknesses in the face of persistent complexities. Few theories fit perfectly. However, this is never a peaceful process.

The radical reinterpretation of current thinking about the ear, which is described below, first caught my attention because of its clinical applicability as therapy.

The role of the human ear

A man clings all his days to what he received in his youth.

Paracelsus

Literature summary:

Searching the literature, and taking the degree of disagreement among specialists as my barometer, it quickly became apparent that the ear is a much studied, yet incompletely understood organ. What follows is a summary of the orthodox views regarding the anatomy, neurophysiology and therapeutic potential of the ear. This information was gathered from my medical school basic science curriculum, a literature search and interviews with specialists in the field.

The human ear has two important functions: hearing with the cochlea and balance with the vestibule. The ear is routinely given short shrift in gross anatomy classes where its tiny intrinsic muscles such as the tensor tympani or the stapedius are rarely seen. In anatomy textbooks, the eighth cranial nerve, the acoustic nerve, routinely gets the least print.

Theoretically, the structural relationship and function of the ossicles involves sound, in the form of vibrational energy, which transverses the ossicles from tympanic membrane to oval window. The ossicles are, in order, the hammer (malleus), the anvil (incus) and the stirrup (stapes). The clinical significance of Rinne's and Webber's signs are presented as determinations of air and bone vibrations conducted to the oval window – the former by the ossicles, the latter by the larger skull bones. Additionally, theory has it that this vibration is transmitted through endolymph fluid in the superior segment of the spiraling cochlea (the vestibular ramp) up past high, middle and low frequency receptors (cells of Corti) to the apex of the spiral cupula, before descending finally via the inferior segment of the cochlea (tympanic ramp) to the round window.

Among the orthodoxy, the only questions remaining are those regarding the processes which transform vibrational wave energy to electrical energy at the cells of Corti, and ultimately to cognitive perception of recognizable sounds at the level of the cortex.

Comparison of orthodox and unorthodox views

1) Regarding the embryological origin of the human ear:

If you want to understand what something is, you must look to see where it came from.

Goethe

Orthodox: It is commonly understood that the ear is divided into three parts: the external ear (meatus and canal), the middle ear (tympanic membrane, ossicles, middle ear muscles) and the inner ear (vestibule and cochlea).

Unorthodox: An appreciation of embryology suggests that there are, practically speaking, only two ears – an external and an internal ear. We know that the embryo originally consists of a series of five branchial arches [3]. The adult ear develops from the first two. More specifically, the first brachial arch will develop into the first two ossicles of the ear (the malleus with its muscle and the incus) and falls under the innervation of the trigeminal nerve (5th cranial nerve). The second brachial arch produces the third ossicle (stapes with its stapedius muscle) and is innervated by the facial nerve (7th cranial nerve). More can be made of the other organs which arise from these first two brachial arches (lower jaw with adductive muscles from the first and upper part of the larynx, the hyoid bone and the anterior ventral segment of the digastric muscle which opposes the jaw adductors) but references must suffice for interested readers [4]. My point here is that the ear is functionally understood as tripartite while actually comprising a polarity. This distinction becomes therapeutically significant in terms of high-frequency audition. (see following)

2) *Sound transmission:*

We really ought to know by now how the ear works.

Ashmore (in *Nature* 8/84)

Orthodox: The commonly accepted role of the external canal as regarding sound transmission is considered to be as a low-frequency filter. It is observed that bone vibrations of the skull can create sound waves in the external canal which excite the tympanic membrane [5]. The role of the ossicles is commonly understood as transmission linking sound vibrations at the tympanic membrane to the oval window [6]. The role of the middle ear muscles, the tensor tympani and the stapedius, according to von Bekesy, is to maintain the connection between ossicles. This long-standing interpretation is currently being challenged by Howell. The role of the endolymph is to further conduct the wave of kinetic energy towards its destination, the cells of Corti. The tectorial membrane's role is to anchor the hairs of the cells of Corti in order to facilitate the shearing force necessary to set up an active potential which will propagate along the eighth cranial nerve to the cortex for cognitive processing. The role of the cochlea is to contain the fluid and its kinetic force thus preserving the sound fidelity. The role of the round window is to dampen kinetic energy [7]

Unorthodox [4]:

A) The distance separating the incus and the stapes, sometimes up to 1 mm, and bridged by collagen, cannot conduct sound with fidelity commensurate with human hearing. To assume that high frequencies can be transmitted intact through this distance and medium seems unreasonable, as rather than transmitting vibratory energy from the external to internal ear, the function of the ossicles is to dampen tympanic membrane vibratory energy via a kinetic negative feedback loop originating at the hyperkinetic endolymph. This fluid force is transmitted to the base of the stapes, then to the incus, and finally to the malleus in order to diminish vibratory sensation headed to the ear. In effect, rather than transmitting sound, the ossicles serve a protective role by dampening excessive vibratory energy transmitted to compact bone at the tympanic sulcus. Although the first, Tomatis is no longer alone in assigning a protective role to the middle ear. (Simmons 1964).

B) Endolymph is always moving [8]. Therefore, to consider that it can carry specific waves amidst the turbulence seems unreasonable. Additionally, the observation that sequential sounds can be transmitted almost instantaneously is inconsistent with the assertion that the sound is transmitted through the fluid [9]. The function of the endolymph as regards hearing is to buffer the shearing potential of the vibrational force. Here in the ear, as in other parts of the body (joints, brain vault), fluid does what fluid does best: its role as endolymph is to absorb kinetic energy and protect contingent structures from damage.

C) Removal of the ossicles in no way diminishes osseous conduction [5]. However, removal of the ossicles would result in a relatively flaccid contact between the tympanic membrane and the tympanic sulcus, thereby accounting for the observed loss of 60db in air conduction.

D) Tomatis claims that osseous conduction (a highly controversial field at this time) is the major route of sound conduction to the inner ear. The route is as follows: air vibration hitting the tympanic membrane is spread outward along its radiating fibers to the tympanic sulcus where the petrous pyramid (compact bone) conducts the kinetic energy directly to the cochlea, and finally to the basilar membrane [4]. A consideration of the anatomy of the tympanic membrane suggests that arciform fibers collect wave impulses and disperse them to the periphery of the membrane, which is firmly attached to the sulcus. Opponents of bone conduction note that only direct contact of the vibration tuning fork to bone yields true fidelity and that the soft tissues atop the skull constitute resistance [5]. In light of that observation, it is interesting to note that the tympanic sulcus is the location where bone receives vibrational energy most directly. Furthermore, the endochondral capsule is the only place in the human body where primitive bone which developed from fetal cartilage persists unchanged (with no resorption) from before birth until after death. Thus, this static medium is the ideal conductor for vibratory energy. (Whales hear via osseous conduction). The oval and round windows, like the Eustachian tube, function as additional buffers against the shearing force requisite in audition. To function optimally, the human ear must maintain a micro-homeostasis which allows for maximal sensory perception with minimal shearing and destruction of hair cells. The role of the middle ear then is to guard the sensitive cells of Corti which are responsible for energy transduction within the inner ear.

E) Flock was not the first to observe that the basilar membrane vibrates. However, he was the first to announce the disruptive observation that hair cells, the organs of Corti, contain actin and a variety of protein associated with contractility [10]. Consequently, the suggestion arises that the cells of Corti are end organs rather than sensory cells, implying that they play a role in cochlear mechanics. Therefore, where once we thought that the endolymph vibrates the basilar membrane, we now have data calling that into question. It remains solely a matter of interpretation as to whether the endolymphatic eddy is the cause of, or, as Tomatis suggests [4], the result of the resonating membrane.

F) The tiny stapedius muscle, which controls the stapes and thereby regulates high-frequency audition, is the only muscle of the human body which never rests [4]. Even the heart pulsates, a motion which involves periodicity and therefore a rest of sorts. The stapedius, however, is constantly involved in regulating sound perception from the fourth month post-conception until the moment of death [11]. This constancy is significant as regards cortical charge.

3) *Ear neurology:*

The Nerves of the Terrible Pterygopalatine Traffic Circle
– every anatomy student's nightmare.

The ear is the Rome of the body. As a student of gross anatomy, it struck me that almost all cranial nerves lead to the ear. Whether directly or anastomatically, (communicating via cross-connections) the ear is involved with cranial nerves 2-11. The 5th and 7th cranial nerves innervate the ossicular muscles. But, in order to fully appreciate the extra-auditory and extra-gyratory role of the acoustic or eighth cranial nerve, we must understand the oculo-cephalo-gyre crossover which, in mammals showing a high degree of cortical sophistication, is apparently under the control of the visual function [4]. It is customary when dealing with cortical functions to link eye, head and neck mobility with the optic nerve. However, the co-ordinated interplay of these functional structures is under the control of the acoustic nerve. This structure, appropriately called the audio-opto-oculo-cephalo-gyro cross-over is the major mechanism of reception and integration of perception. Therefore, the ear is now understood to be neurologically involved with the optic or 2nd cranial nerve, the oculomotor or 3rd cranial nerve, the trochlear or 4th cranial nerve, the abducens or 6th cranial nerve and the spinal-accessory or 11th cranial nerve, which is responsible for posterior-lateral musculature of the neck.

Not satisfied with this scope of neurological involvement, the ear has a fascinating tie into the 10th cranial nerve or the vagus, "path of the wandering soul." What has the vagus to do with the ear? For those of us who think of the tympanic membrane solely as a receiver for sound waves, it is instructive to recollect that a solitary cutaneous sensory antenna from the vagus presents on its outer surface and that its inner surface is sensitized by the vagus via an anastomosis with the glosso-pharyngeal or 9th cranial nerve. What is the significance of vagal and acoustic interaction? Let us track this path throughout the body. The vagus wanders on contacting next the postural back muscles via an anastomosis with the spino-accessory or 11th cranial nerve, then sensitizes that part of the larynx responsible for vocalization via the upper laryngeal nerve, before delivering motor innervation via the recurrent laryngeal nerves. Subsequently, the vagus innervates the bronchi and heart before joining the opposing vagal nerve and diving through the diaphragm to innervate the entire viscera including the gastro-intestinal tract from esophagus to anus (via anastomosis with sacral nerves 2, 3, and 4).

The effect which audition has via the vagus is substantial. Prasad observed cardiac depression upon syringing the ear [12]. But this ought not surprise us. What would a scary movie be without the emotionally manipulative sound track? Think of the effect which a patient in the process of vomiting has on our own intestinal homeostasis. It is empathy, or perhaps direct vagal stimulation from our tympanic membrane to our gastrointestinal track which evokes our similar contraction. As the ear becomes appreciated as our primary sensory organ (for both internal and external phenomenon) as well as a vagally mediated internal moderator via its extensive anastomotic innervations, a theoretical basis for audio-therapy comes into focus.

This is only a glimpse of some major reinterpretations of ear structure and function. The bibliography offers the reader the opportunity to pursue these and other equally challenging assertions in greater detail than the scope of this report justifies.

The work of Dr. Alfred A. Tomatis

Creative imagination is frequently associated with the interplay between two conceptual frameworks.

Koestler

Born in 1920, Dr. Tomatis earned his M.D. from the Faculte de Paris before specializing in oto-rhino-laryngology. En route to establishing the International Association of audio-Psycho-Phonology, Dr. Tomatis was distinguished as follows: Chevalier de la Sante Publique (Knight of Public Health) 1951; Medaille d'Or de la Recherche Scientifique (Gold Medal for Scientific Research) 1958; Grande Medaille de Vermeil de la Ville de Paris 1962; Prix Clemence Isaure 1967, Medaille d'Or de la Societé Arts, Science et Lettres 1968; et Commandeur de Merite Culturel et Artistique 1970.

As a scientist, Tomatis is well recognized for his experimental breakthroughs in the field of auditory neurophysiology. For example, while treating hearing impaired factory workers by day, and scotoma-cursed opera singers by night, Tomatis noticed a similarity of symptoms between the two patient populations. After further investigation, he formulated the law describing the feedback loop between the larynx and the ear: "the larynx emits only the range that the ear controls." In other words, one can reproduce vocally only those sounds which one can hear. This discovery was recognized by the Academy of Sciences of Paris and the French Academy of Medicine who, in 1957, announced the Tomatis Effect in honor of its discoverer.

As a clinician, Tomatis has achieved a reputation for successful and unorthodox therapies whose scope exceeded the scope of oto-rhino-laryngology. The list of maladies successfully treated via high-frequency auditive therapy includes: *Ear, Nose and Throat disorders:* (hearing and voice loss [13], stuttering [14], tinnitus [15], otitis media [15], scotomas [16, 17]); *Neurological disorders:* (toe walking from vestibular nuclei problems [18], drooling [15, 19], strabismus

[15]); *Psychiatric disorders:* (depression [20], attention deficit disorder [21], hyperactivity [21]); and *Learning disorders:* (dyslexia [22], inability to concentrate [15]); and a variety of balance/co-ordination problems related to the ear's vestibular disorders [15]. These therapeutic coups occur via retraining the ear muscles using another Tomatis invention, the electronic ear (see below). These claims regarding the therapeutic efficacy of filtered sound were what drew me to France. What follows will be a brief description of the theoretical bases and practical applications of Tomatis's therapeutic work.

Electronic Ear and middle ear micro-gymnastics:

This machine trains athletes of the middle ear – it produces champion listeners.

Tomatis

Theory:

Most of us have fiddled with the bass/treble knob on a stereo set. What we probably did not recognize, however, was that it was easier to hear the bass sounds than it was the treble ones. (Bass is closer to touch on the continuum of sensible vibratory energy, that is, hearing as tactile reception is a form of touch). This difference in relative ease of listening became the crux of Dr. Tomatis's Electronic Ear. This machine is designed to help the ear acquire three functions: listening, monitoring of language and laterality.

The Electronic Ear works by delivering to the listener's ear a course of sound which is progressively filtered along a continuum from normal non-filtered sound to sound where all save frequencies greater than 8000 hz have been filtered away. In addition, the sound delivered to the patient varies its pitch between treble and bass sounds, according to specific acoustic dynamics. Consequently, the stapedius muscle must control the stapes in order to listen to ascending high-frequency sounds as well as accommodate the fluctuations between bass and treble at the given frequency. This challenge to the atrophied middle ear muscles (especially the stapedius muscle of the stapes which is primarily responsible for high-frequency discrimination) constitutes the micro-gymnastics, which orchestrate the reattainment of the physiologic listening or focusing function of the ear.

Application:

Auditory disorders are easily identified by noticing aberrations from normal listening posture (note monastic posture of head inclined at 30 degrees which levels the horizontal semi-circular canal), atonality or lifeless speech, poor body tonus, substandard motor co-ordination, facial dyskinesias and lateralization to the left (talking out of left side of mouth). Predictors of auditory disorders involving high frequencies would include dyslexics, stutterers (i.e. a variety of learning disabled people) as well as products of traumatic births (caesarian sections, premature, forceps-damaged, and anoxic as well as occasional twin births) [24].

Tomatis is given credit for being the first to appreciate the important neuro-physiological distinction between hearing and listening. The former is non-selective, whereas the latter is a focusing of the ears and an attending to one of the many sounds that are heard simultaneously. Hearing is less strenuous than listening, which involves will power. Tomatis's listening test differs from the audiogram of the audiologist in that the listening test is concerned not only with the organic capacities of the ear, but also with the degree to which the ear's potential is being utilized by the patient. An audiologist will frustratedly acknowledge that many people come to them with hearing problems who, according to their audiograms, can hear perfectly well. In fact, their problem is not with hearing, but with listening. A course of therapy with the Electronic Ear has been shown to improve these listening problems as measured by reattainment of optimum air and bone conduction curves on a standard audiogram.

Equally exciting is the ability of geriatric patients with high-frequency hearing loss to attain partial or complete recovery of their optimum audiometric curves. In fact, Tomatis has demonstrated therapeutic successes in all types of hearing loss cases save sensorineural loss as measured by standard audiographic analysis.

Laterality:

*My left hand hath laid the foundations of the earth
and my right hand hath spanned the heavens.*

Isaiah 48:13

Theory:

Who can explain the phenomenon of asymmetry in our nervous system? No one has yet. Who can offer insight into its significance? Tomatis's work on laterality as a consequence of this asymmetry is compelling. Aside from the stapedial workout designed to aid the reattainment of high-frequency audition, Tomatis's Electronic Ear trains the right ear to be the dominant or leading ear. The basis for this dextrophilia is an understanding of the asymmetrical auditory pathways [25]. According to Tomatis, the left hemisphere's speech center (Broca) is most directly connected with the right ear [4]. Furthermore, the right recurrent laryngeal nerve (connected via the right vagus to the right ear), in looping under the right subclavian artery, constitutes a significantly shorter pathway than that of the left recurrent laryngeal nerve which loops under the aorta. Consequently, significantly longer auditory feedback loop exists on the left compared to the right side of the body. Furthermore, an individual with a dominant left ear must process auditory information over a significantly longer transcerebral auditory pathways (left ear to right auditory center to left auditory center to organs of speech = 70-140 m) than is required by a right-dominant listener (right ear to left auditory center to organs of speech = 30-60 cm) [15,26].

Application:

The process of lateralization to the right, achieved through the delivery of sound increasingly to the right ear, has the effect of facilitating and accelerating the patient's processing of sensory and cognitive information [4].

This lateralization is an essential aspect of the therapeutic ear training which has proven valuable to the variety of patients listed above.

Sonic Rebirth and uterine hearing:

... Hence, in a season of calm weather,
Through inland far we be,
Our souls have sight of that immortal sea
Which brought us hither.
Can in a moment travel thither,
And see the children sport upon the shore,
And hear the mighty waters rolling evermore.

Wordsworth from "Intimations of Immortality"

Theory:

Perhaps Tomatis's most provocative theory involves the idea of fetal audition [27]. Today, thirty years after Tomatis postulated this phenomenon, investigation of fetal audition is in vogue. However, despite a rash of recent studies, it remains solely a matter of speculation whether the fetus can hear, and if so, what the fetus hears. We know that the acoustic nerve is fully myelinated and functioning at 4.5 months post-conception [15] and we also know that the fetal eustachian tube is patent, thereby permitting contact to the inner ear via embryonic fluid [4]. Tomatis suggests that the fetus hears the maternal heart and respiration as well as her intestinal gurgling. This, he postulates, comprises a constant background noise. It is important as cortical charge (see below) and may be the source of our collective attraction to the sound of surf or of our inborn sense of rhythm. The fetus would hear this biological noise, but to what would it listen? What is the only sound which comes and goes at irregular intervals? The voice of the mother. According to Tomatis, only the voice of the mother can penetrate via her bones (see osseous conduction) to the intrauterine world. The child's attention is fixed on this irregular sound which may serve as the fetus's first target of communication. Studies show that the newborn responds preferentially to the voice of the mother [28]. Pediatricians have observed that the newborn demonstrates preference for the mother's voice [28]. What is a reasonable explanation for this observation? Intrauterine hearing is a possibility.

Applications:

The practical application of this theory are intriguing. By taking a uterine and birth history of a person with an auditory disorder, the therapist is able to predict a very curious event. Certain sound frequencies corresponding to intrauterine audition will evoke unpleasant sensations in adult listeners whose mothers experienced trauma at a certain gestational period. Additionally, a variety of neuroses are ameliorated simply by following a course called sonic rebirth. This involves, in part, the passage from audition through a simulated liquid element, to audition through an atmospheric element. The mother's voice is recorded (often reading a child's story) and presented to the patient over a period of weeks progressively filtered from 8000 hz to 100 hz thereby simulating the auditory experience of uterine existence, labor, birth and reunion, this time via atmospheric conduction, with the child listening to the maternal voice while nestled in the mother's arms. Freud's psychoanalytic theories and practice were once considered equally bizarre. Unlike Freud's cases, however, the patients of Tomatis who undergo sonic rebirth are objectively evaluated both behaviorally and using audiograms, which assume a motivational and co-operative component.

One fascinating spin-off of the sonic rebirth is its application in learning a foreign language. For example, a businessman who wants to learn Arabic before being transferred to that country would undergo a sonic rebirth while listening to a course of filtered Arabic. In this way, his ears are progressively sensitized to the idiosyncratic sounds of that language. Without his ears being able to distinguish particular sounds, certainly his tongue would not be able to pronounce these sounds (remember the Tomatis Effect). In this manner, Tomatis has had extraordinary success giving people a new "mother tongue" in a language of their choice [29].

Primacy of the ear:

The ear builds, organizes and nourishes the nervous system.

Tomatis [15]

Theory:

Tomatis asserts that the brain receives more stimuli via the ears than from any other organ. He considers skin to be differentiated ear rather than visa versa. In his two volume work, *Towards a Human Listening*, [4], he builds an intriguing defense of this radical departure from orthodoxy which involves, for example, phylogenetic data suggesting, paradoxically, that the ear preceded the nervous system. Furthermore, an impressive case is made suggesting that our sense corpuscles (Meissners, Pacinian, Krause, Merkel's) are differentiated organs of Corti. (See Flock et al, [10] regarding the recent confusion about the nature of the organ of Corti). Whether one emerges from a review of Tomatis's *Towards a Human Listening* surprised or not, certainly one gains an appreciation of the hitherto underrated role of the ear.

Application:

An understanding of the idiosyncratic physiological aspects of the human ear has important therapeutic applications. Tinnitus, for example, is a debilitating hearing disorder whose etiology is undetermined and whose treatment (masking) is inadequate [28]. Tomatis asserts that tinnitus results from a swollen inner ear artery against which sympathomimetic drugs are ineffective. This is so, he explains, because of all the arteries in the human body, this artery is not under sympathetic control [15]. Tinnitus is only one of many problematic maladies which Tomatis treats successfully using an appreciation of the peculiarities of the human ear and a course of high-frequency auditive therapy via his invention, the Electronic Ear.

Cortical charge:

There are sounds which are as good a pick-me-up as two cups of coffee.

Tomatis [15]

Theory:

The most exciting theory of Tomatis, and the one which led me to consider the role of sacred music as therapy, is the concept of cortical charge. Experience tells us that some sounds put us to sleep (lullabies) and some keep us awake (traffic); some calm us down (surf on the beach) and some make us dance all night (rhythm). A hard driving beat practically forces us to tap our feet. The screech of chalk on blackboard makes us scream and contract in discomfort. We are constantly bathed by sound and Tomatis has devoted his career to analyzing the effect which various components of sound exert on our physiology. The claim that music exerts a profound effect on us is beyond question. What remains is only to establish the correlations, perhaps psychosomatic, perhaps vagally innervated, of these sound components to our physiology. Let us listen to Dr. Tomatis directly. In a lecture before the International Kodaly Symposium in Paris, 1978, he describes cortical charge as follows:

> *The ear is primarily an apparatus intended to provide a cortical charge in terms of electric potential. In fact, sound is transformed into nervous influx by the coliform cells of the cochlear-vestibular apparatus. The charge of energy obtained from the influx of nervous impulses reaches the cortex, which then distributes it*

throughout the body toning up the whole system and imparting greater dynamism to the human being.

All sounds cannot effect this process of charging. I pointed out that on the basilar membrane the ciliform cells of Corti are much more densely packed in the part reserved for the perception of high frequencies than in the one where the low frequencies are distributed; so that the transmission of energy that is caught up towards the cortex is much more intense when it comes from the zone of the high frequencies than when it comes from the part reserved for the low frequencies.

Thus the high sounds supply a more concentrated nervous influx and thus increase the effect of charging. This is the reason why I called the sounds rich in high harmonics the "charging sounds," in opposition to the low sounds or "dis-charging sounds." These low sounds supply insufficient energy to the cortex, which may even exhaust the individual, so much that they conduct corporal motor responses which actually, in themselves, absorb more energy than the labyrinth can furnish. The implication of this fact at the psycho-dynamic level explains that a depressed person tends to direct his hearing more intensively towards low frequencies which are the sonic range of visceral life: she actually becomes more aware of the noise of her breathing, of her heartbeat, and so on. It seems as if her ear has lost its ability to be used as an "antenna" for communication; instead, it is directed to the inside life.

The aim will be to provoke, with sonic training made of high-frequencies heard in a listening posture, this cortical charge to energize the individual. The effects of the training generally manifest themselves in the following ways to the subject:

- greater motivation and competence in working
- lower susceptibility to fatigue
- awareness of dynamism
- better possibilities of attention and concentration
- better memorization.

Application:

Anecdotal evidence suggests that certain high-frequency sounds confer alertness and stamina to the listener, thereby enhancing performance. For example, students report that listening to Gregorian chants or classical music increases their ability to concentrate. If this modus operandi sounds strange to the reader, consider the time honored prescription "whistle while you work." Or try to imagine a military marching band without the fife. Granted the drums would discourage any waltzing by enforcing the left-right-left-right, but without the fife producing a cortical charge, how great would one's endurance be? Bugles, bagpipes…always the high-frequency tones are found en route to battle. Perhaps these shrill high-frequency tones impart an enthusiasm via neurophysiologically mediated cortical charge.

Who is Dr. Weeks?

Bradford S. Weeks, M.D. is a pioneer in corrective medicine and psychiatry whose practice involves helping people make corrections of various imbalances on their physical, vital, emotional and spiritual levels of life.

He appreciates all effective, cost-effective and safe modalities for caring and uses prescription medications only in optimal doses. His practice has focused on caring for patients dealing with cancer, chronic degenerative neurologic diseases (Alzheimer's, MS and Parkinson's) as well as various psychiatric/metabolic disorders (schizophrenia, manic depression, depression, obesity, diabetes). He is also a beekeeper and a world-renowned expert in the medicinal use of honeybee products.

He and his wife, Laura, currently deliver care at their Corrective Health Clinic on Whidbey Island off the coast of Washington State, USA. For more information visit http://weeksmd.com

References:

1 McCandless, G., 'Hearing Aids and Auditory Rehabilitation,' 1981, in English, G.M. [ed] *Otolaryngology Loose Leaf Series*, Harper & Row, Vol. 2, Chapter 52, Philadelphia, 1986.

2 Michelson, R., 'Electrical Stimulation of the Cochlea,' 1979, in English, G.M., [ed] *Otolaryngology Loose Leaf Series*, Vol. 1, Chapter 57, Harper & Row, Philadelphia, 1986.

3 Pearson, A., 'Developmental Anatomy of the Ear,' 1978, in English, G.M. [ed] *Otolaryngology Loose Leaf Series*, Vol. 1, Chapter 1, Harper & Row, Philadelphia, 1986.

4 Tomatis, A., *Vers L'Ecoute Humaine*, Editions ESF, Paris 1974.

5 Tonndorf, J., 'Bone Conduction,' In Tobias, J.V., [ed] *Foundations of Modern Auditory Theory*, Vol. 2, Academic Press, New York, 1972, p.200.

6 Moller, A., 'The Middle Ear,' In Tobias J.V. [ed] *Foundations of Modern Auditory Theory*, Vol. 2, Academic Press, New York, 1972, p.135.

7 Nuttall, A., & Ross, M., 'Auditory Physiology,' 1980, in English, G.M., [ed] *Otolaryngology Loose Leaf Series*, Vol 1, Chapter 3, Harper & Row, Philadelphia, 1986.

8 Juhn, S., 'Biochemistry of the Inner and Middle Ear,' 1983, in English, G.M., [ed] *Otolaryngology Loose Leaf Series*, Vol. 1, Chapter 60, Harper & Row, Philadelphia, 1986.

9 Fritze, W. & Kohler, W., 'Frequency Composition of Spontaneous Cochlear Emissions,' *Arch. Otol.*, 242, (1) 1985, pp.43-8.

10 Flock, A., *Hearing – Physiological Bases and Psycho-physics* [ed. Klinke] Springer, Berlin, 1983.

11 Howell, P., 'Are Two Muscles Needed for the Normal Functioning of the Mammalian Ear?' *Acta Otol* (Stockh), 98, 1984, pp.204-7.

12 Prasad, K., 'Cardiac depression on Syringing the Ear,' *J. Laryngol Otol.*, 98 (10) Oct. 1984, p.1013.

13 Tomatis, A., *La Voix Chantee – sa Physiologie – sa Pathologie – sa Reeducation*, Cours de L'Hopital Bichat, March 1960.

14 Tomatis, A., Recherches sur la Pathologie de Begaiement, *Journal Francais d'Oto-Rhino-Laryngologie*, Vol. 3, No. 4, p.384, 1954.

15 Taped interview with Tomatis, Paris, August, 1986.

16 Tomatis, A., 'La reeducation de la Voix – Les different Methodes de Traitement,' *La Vie Medicale*, No. 20, May 1974.

17 Tomatis, A., *Correction de la Voix Chantee*, Cours international de Phonologie, Libraire Maloine. pp.335-353, 1953.

18 Tomatis, A., 'Les Bases Neuro-physiologiques de la Musicotherapie,' *Bulletin de ISME*, Conservatoire de Grenoble, April, 1974.

19 Grewal, D. et. al., 'Transtympanic Neurectomies for Control of Drooling,' *Auris Nasus Larynx*, 11(2) 1984, pp.109-14.

20 Tomatis, A., 'La Musicotherapie et les Depressiones Nerveuses,' Rapport au IV Congres Int'l d'Audio-Psycho-Phonologie, Madrid, 1974.

21 Le Gall, A., *Le redressement de Certains Deficiencies Psychologiques et Psycol-Pedagogiques*, Inspecteur general de L'Instruction Publique, Paris, March 1961.

22 Tomatis, A., *Dyslexie*, Cours a L'Ecole d'Anthropologie, Editions Soditap, 1967.

23 Lafon, R., *Vocabulaire de Psychopedagogie*, P.U.F., Paris.

24 Tomatis, A., *Education et Dyslexie*, Editions ESF, Paris, 1972.

25 Gacek, R., 'Neuroanatomy of the Auditory System,' In Tobias J.V. [ed] *Foundations of Modern Auditory Theory*, Vol 2, Academic Press, New York, 1972, p.239.

26 Le Gall, A., *Le Redressement de Certains Deficiences Psychologiques et Psycho-Pedagogiques*, Inspecteur General de L'Instruction Publique, Paris, March 1961.

27 Tomatis, A., *La Nuit Uterine*, Editions Stock, Paris 1981.

28 DeCasper, A. & Fifer, W., 'Of Human Bonding – Newborns Prefer Their Mother's Voices,' *Science*, 208, 1980, pp.1174-6.

29 Tomatis, A., 'L'Electronique au Service des Langues Vivantes,' *Bulletin de L'Union des Ass. des Anciens Eleves des Lycees et Colleges Francais,* March 1960.

30 Vernon, J., 'Relief of Tinnitus by Masking Treatment,' 1982 in English, G.M., [ed] *Otolaryngology Loose Leaf Series*, Vol. 1, Chapter 53, Harper & Row, Philadelphia, 1986.

31 Prou, J., *Le Chant Gregorien et la Sanctification des Fideles*, V111 Congres International de Music Sacree, Rome 1985.

Bibliography for Appendix:

Albert, M., *Clinical Neurology of Aging*, Oxford Uni. Press, New York, 1984.

Bannatyne, A., *Reading: An Auditory Vocal Process*, Academic Therapy Publications, San Rafael, Ca., U.S., 1973.

Clifford, T., *Tibetan Buddhist Medicine and Psychiatry,* Weiser Pub. Inc., 1984.

Dhonden, Y. MD., *Health Through Balance*, [ed. and trans. Hopkins], Snow Lion Publications, Ithaca, NY., 1986.

Gacek, R., 'The Vestibular System,' in English, G.M., [ed] *Otolaryngology Loose Leaf Series,* Harper & Row, Philadelphia, 1979.

Gilmor, T, *Overview of the Tomatis Method*, Ontario Psychological Association, Listening Center Pub., Toronto, Canada, 1982.

Gilmor, T, *Participant Characteristics and Follow-Up Evaluations of Participants in the Listening Training Program, 1978-1983*, Listening Center Pub., Toronto, Canada, 1984.

Gilmor, T, *Application of the Listening Training Program in the School,* Listening Center Pub., Toronto, Canada, 1984.

Hammil, D. and Larsen, S., 'The Relationship of Selected Auditory Perceptual Skills and Reading Ability,' *Journal of Learning Disabilities*, Vol. 7, 1974.

Harrer, H., *Seven Years in Tibet*, Vol. 1, Chapter 8, Pan Books Ltd. London, 1982 Row, 1986.

Hudspeth, A., 'The Cellular Basis of Hearing: The Biophysics of Hair Cells,' *Science,* Vol. 230, No. 4727, 11/15/85, p.745.

Kuhn, T., *The Structure of Scientific Revolutions*, Uni. of Chicago Press, Chicago, 1962.

Le Feuvre, L., *Le Chant Gregorien*, Pub. Abbaye Sainte-Anne de Kergonan, Phouharnel, France, 1986.

Madaule, P., *Audio-Psycho-Phonology for Singers and Musicians*, Potchefstrom University, South Africa, Listening Center Pub., Toronto, Canada, 1976.

Moushegian, G; Rupert, A; and Whitcomb, M., 'Processing of Auditory Information by Medial Superior-Olivary Neurons,' in Tobias, J.V. [ed]: *Foundations of Modern Auditory Theory,* Vol. 2, Academic Press, New York, 1972, p.263.

Quick, C., 'Ototoxicity,' in English, G.M., [ed] *Otolaryngology Loose Leaf Series,* Vol. 1, Harper & Row, Philadelphia, 1986.

Russell, J. and Sellick, P., in *J. Physiol.*, Vol. 284, London, 1978, p.261.

Stutt, H., 'The Tomatis Method: A Review of Current Research,' Unpublished manuscript, McGill University, 1983.

Tomatis, A., 'Music Filtree et Pedagogie Psycho-Sensorielle chez les Enfants Presentant des Troubles de la Communication,' 3rd Congres Int'l d'Audio-Psycho-Phonologie; Anvers, Belgium, 1973.

von Bekesy, G., *Experiments in Hearing*, McGraw Hill, NY, 1960.

For Sound Therapy product information see last page. Bibliography is on next page.

Bibliography

1. 'A Report of the Task Force on the National Strategic Research Plan,' National Institute on Deafness and other Communication Disorders, National Institutes of Health, Bethesda, Maryland, April 1989, p. 74.

2. Access Economics, 2006, *The Economic Impact and Cost of Hearing Loss in Australia,* CRC Hear and the Victorian Deaf Society.

3. Anastasio, T. J., and Patton, P. E., 'A Two-Stage Unsupervised Learning Algorithm Reproduces Multisensory Enhancement in a Neural Network Model of the Corticotectal System,' *The Journal of Neuroscience,* 23(17) July 30, 2003, pp.6713-6727.

4. Baguley, D. M; Humphriss, R. L; Axon, P.R; and Moffat, D. A., 'The Clinical Characteristics of Tinnitus in Patients with Vestibular Schwannoma,' *Skull Base,* 16(2) May 2006, pp.49–58. Prepublished online 2006 February 13. doi: 10.1055/s-2005-926216.PMCID: PMC1502033

5. Berendt, Joachim. E., *The Third Ear,* Henry Holt and Company Inc., New York, 1992.

6. Birnholz J.C. et al., 'The development of human fetal hearing,' *Science,*Vol. 222, 1983, pp.516-518.

7. Blackman, L., *Lucy's Story: Autism and Other Adventures,* Book In Hand, Brisbane, 1999.

8. Campbell, D., *The Mozart Effect,* Hodder and Stoughton, New York, 1997.

9. Cohen, L. et al., 'Psychological Adjusment and Sleep Quality in a Randomised Trial of the Effects of a Tibetan Yoga Intervention in Patients with Lymphoma,' *Cancer,* Vol. 100, No.10, 2004, pp.2253-2260.

10. Clayton A.E. et al, 'Association between osteoporosis and otosclerosis in women,' *Journal of Laryngology & Otology,* Vol.118, No.8, Royal Society of Medicine Press, 2004, pp.617-621.

11. Creagh, S., 'Why I ... use sound therapy,' *Sydney Morning Herald,* October 14, 2004. Cited on 9th Sept 2009: http://www.smh.com.au/articles/2004/10/14/1097607348327. html?from=moreStories

12. Crumpler, Diana, *Chemical Crisis,* Newham, Australia, Scribe Publications, 1994.

13. De Chicchisa, E. R. et al, 'Vitamin D and calcium deficiency initiated in pregnancy and maintained after weaning accelerate auditory dysfunction in the offspring in BALB/cJ mice,' *Nutrition Research,* Vol. 26, Issue 9, Sept. 2006, pp.486-491.

14. Doige, N., *The Brain that Changes Itself,* Scribe Publications, Carlton North, Vic, 2008.

15. Dougherty, R.F; et al., 'Dichotic pitch: a new stimulus distinguishes normal and dyslexic auditory function,' *Neuro Report, Auditory and Vestibular Systems,* Vol. 9, Issue 13, 14 Sept. 1998, pp.3001-3005.

16. Eccles, John C., *The Human Mystery,* The Gifford Lectures, University of Edinburgh, 1977–78.

17. 'Environmental Impact on Hearing: Is Anyone Listening?' *Environmental Health Perspectives* Vol. 102, No. 12, Dec. 1994. cited on 31 Aug. 2009: http://www.ehponline. org/docs/1994/102-11/focus2.html

18. Freeman S; Sichel JY; Sohmer H., 'Bone conduction experiments in animals – evidence for a non-osseous mechanism,' *Hearing Research,* Vol.146, 2000, pp.72-80. Cited on: http://onderwijs1.amc.nl/medfysica/doc/Bone%20conduction.htm

19. Froehling DA; Bowen J.M; et al., 'The canalith repositioning procedure for the treatment of benign paroxysmal positional vertigo: a randomized controlled trial,' Mayo Clinic Proceedings. 75(7) 2000, pp.695-700.
Cited on 9th August 2009, from *Vertigo: Its Causes and Treatment,* Huai Y. Cheng, M.D., http://www.thedoctorwillseeyounow.com/articles/other/vertigo_17/

20. Gerristen, J., 'A Review of Research done on Tomatis Auditory Stimulation,' http://www.

tomatis.com/English/Articles/research.htm

21. Gilmor, T.M; Madaule, P; & Thompson, B.M. (eds) *About The Tomatis Method,* the Listening Centre Press, Toronto, 1989.

22. Gilmor, T. 'The Efficacy of the Tomatis Method for Children with Learning and Communication Disorders; A Meta Analysis,' *International Journal of Listening,* Vol. 13, 1999, pp.12-23.

23. Golden, I., 'Homoeoprophylaxis – a Proven Alternative to Vaccination,' *Nourished Magazine,* Dec 2008. Cited on Sept 7th 2009 on: http://nourishedmagazine.com.au/ blog/articles/homoeoprophylaxis-%E2%80%93-a-proven-alternative-to-vaccination

24. Golz A; Fradis M; Martzu D; Netzer A; and Joachims H.Z., 'Stapedius muscle myoclonus,' *Ann Otol Rhinol Laryngol* 112(6) 2003, pp.522-4. Cited on http://www. dizziness-and-balance.com/disorders/hearing/tinnitus.htm

25. Grandjean, P; Landrigan, P., 'Developmental neurotosicity of industrial chemicals,' *The Lancet,* Vol. 368, Issue 9553, pp.2167-2178.

26. Gray, H. *Gray's Anatomy,* Fifteenth edition, Barnes and Noble, USA, 1995.

27. Greenfield, Susan. *The Human Brain,* Phoenix, London, 1997.

28. Gupta, M.S., 'Neurodevelopmental Disorders in Children – Autism and ADHD,' EnvironmentalChemistry.com. April 14, 2008. Accessed on-line: 8/26/2009 http://EnvironmentalChemistry.com/yogi/environmental/200804childrenautismadhd. html

29. Han, B. I.; Lee, H.W; Kim, T.Y; Lim, J. S; and Shin, K. S; 'Tinnitus: Characteristics, Causes, Mechanisms, and Treatments,' *J Clin Neurol,* 5(1) March, 2009, pp.11–19. Published online 2009 March 31. doi: 10.3988/jcn.2009.5.1.11. PMCID: PMC2686891

30. Hari, R. and Kiesila, P., 'Deficit of temporal auditory processing in dyslexic adults,' Low Temperature Laboratory, Helsinki University of Technology, 02150, Espoo, Finland, March 1999.

31. Harrison, R.V., 'Representing the Acoustic World within the Brain: Normal and Abnormal Development of Frequency Maps in the Auditory System,' Conference Keynote Address. Proceedings of the 2nd International Conference Sponsored by Phonak.

32. Hazel, J., 'Things that go Bump in the Night,' From *ITHS Newsletter,* 5 Jan 2003.

33. Hess, W. R., *The Biology of the Mind,* the University of Chicago Press, 1964.

34. Hilary, E., *Children of a Toxic Harvest,* Lothian, Melbourne, 1997.

35. Hillecke, T. K; Nickel A. K; Bolay, H.V., 'Scientific Perspectives of Music Therapy,' *Annals of the New York Academy of Sciences,* 1060, 2005, pp.271-282.

36. Hoshino, Y. et al., 'Blood Serotonin and Free Tryptophan Concentration in Autistic Children,' *Neuropsychobiology,* 11, 1984, pp.22-27.

37. *Human Brain,* Princeton University Press, 1975.

38. 'Introduction to the Listening Test, Observations made during the third International Congress of Audio-Psycho-Phonology,' Auver, 1973, in a question-and-answer session with Dr. A. A. Tomatis.

39. 'Investigating the Environmental Origins of Autism,' July 8, 2008, see http://www.scientificamerican.com/article.cfm?id=investigating-environmental-origins-of-autism

40. Jones, E. G; and Powell, T. P. S., 'An Anatomical Study of Converging Sensory Pathways Within The Cerebral Cortex of the Monkey,' *Brain* 93, 1970, pp.793-820. http://brain. oxfordjournals.org/cgi/pdf_extract/93/4/793

41. Joudry, R, *Why Aren't I Learning?* Sound Therapy International, Sydney, 2004.

42. Juhn, S.K; Hunder, B. A; Odland, R. M., 'Blood Labyrinth Barrier and Fluid Dynamics of the Inner Ear,' *Int. Tinnitus Journal,* 7(2) 2001, pp.72-83.

43. Klockhoff, I., 'Impedance fluctuation and a "tensor tympani" syndrome,' In: *Proceedings*

of 4th International Symposium on Acoustic Impedance Measurements, edited by Penha and Pizarro, Universidade Nove de Lisboa, 1981, pp. 69-76. facsimile on www.tinnitus.org

44. Kranowitz, C. S., *The Out of Synch Child,* Penguin, NewYork, 1998.

45. Kuppersmith, R. B. 'Eustachian tube function and dysfunction,' Grand Rounds Archive, Baylor College of Medicine, July 11, 1996. Cited on 13th Sept 2009: http://www.bcm. edu/oto/grand/71196.html

46. Lai, H., and Good, M., 'Music Improves Sleep Quality in Older Adults,' *Journal of Advanced Nursing,* 53(1) January 2006, pp.134-144.

47. Lazar, S., 'Meditation Found to Increase Brain Size,' *Harvard University Gazette,* Jan 23, 2005. Cited on 14 Sept, 2009: http://www.harvardscience.harvard.edu/medicine-health/ articles/meditation-found-increase-brain-size

48. Le Gall, André, *The Adjustment of Certain Psychological and Psycho-Pedagogical Deficiencies with Tomatis Effect Apparatus. The Tomatis Centre,* Paris, March 1961.

49. LePage, Eric L. and Murray, Narelle M., 'Latent cochlear damage in personal stereo users: a study based on click-evoked otoacoustic emissions,' *MJA,* 169, 1998, pp.588-592.

50. Luke, T.C, and Kalpana P., 'Nutritional and Environmental Approaches to Preventing and Treating Autism and Attention Deficit Hyperactivity Disorder (ADHD): A Review,' *The Journal of Alternative and Complementary Medicine,* 14(1) January/February 2008, pp.79-85.

51. Madsen, Lee, and Olle, 'Growing Threats: Toxic Flame Retardants and Children's Health,' Environment California Research and Policy Center March, 2003. Cited on 24th Aug 09: http://www.mindfully.org/Plastic/Flame/Children-Flame-RetardantsMar03.htm

52. Maisch, D; Rapley, B; Rowland, R.E; Podd, J., 'Chronic Fatigue Syndrome – Is prolonged exposure to environmental level powerline frequency electromagnetic fields a co-factor to consider in treatment?' *Journal of the Australasian College of Nutritional & Environmental Medicine,* Vol. 17, No. 2, December 1998, pp. 29-35.

53. Madaule, P., 'Down's Syndrome: Becoming Just One of The Kids,' Originally presented at the meeting of the Association for Down Syndrome of Mexico City, 1989.

54. Maudale, Paul, 'The Dyslexified World', in *About the Tomatis Method,* edited by Gilmor, T. M; Madaule, P; and Thompson, B., The Listening Centre Press, Toronto, Canada, 1989.

55. Maudale, P. *When Listening comes Alive. A Guide to Effective Learning and Communication,* Moulin, Norval, Ontario, Canada, 1994.

56. Minor, L. B., et al., 'Dehiscence of Bone Overlying the Superior Canal as a Cause of Apparent Conductive Hearing Loss,' *Otology & Neurotology:* Vol. 24, Issue 2, March 2003, pp 270-278.

57. Moore, D. R; Rothholtz, V; and King, A. J., 'Hearing: Cortical Activation Does Matter,' *Current Biology,* Vol. 11, Issue 19, 2001, pp.R782-R784.

58. Morse, G., 'Changes in Meniere's Disease Responses as a Function of the Menstrual Cycle.' Cited on 9th August 2009: http://oto2.wustl.edu/men/mn8.htm

59. Moss, K, 'Hearing and Vision Loss Associated with Down Syndrome, TSBVI Deafblind Outreach: http://www.deafblind.com/downmoss.html

60. Motluk, A., 'Meditation Builds up the Brain,' *New Scientist,* 15 November 2005. Cited on 11 Sept 2009: http://www.newscientist.com/search?rbauthors=Alison+Motluk

61. Noble, B., 'Tinnitus and Clinical Psychology,' *Audinews,* 49(6/3) 2006.

62. Ostrander, S; & Schroeder, L., *Superlearning 2000,* Souvenir Press, London, 1996.

63. Parracho, H. et al., 'Differences between the gut microflora of children with autistic spectrum disorders and that of healthy children,' *J. Med Microbiol.,* Vol.54, 2005, pp.987-991.

64. Penfield, Wilder, *The Mystery of the Mind, a Critical Study of Consciousness and the Human Brain,* Princeton University Press, 1975.

65. Ramirez, et al, 'Tensor Tympani Muscle: Strange Chewing Muscle,' *Med. Oral Patol. Oral Cir. Bucal,* 12, 2007, pp.96-100.

66. Richards, G; Richards, P.J; and Joudry, R., 'The Therapeutic Effects of High Band Pass Classical Music and Antioxidant Supplements,' Presented to Australian Audiological Society Conference, Brisbane, 2004. Cited on www.SoundTherapyInternational.com/research

67. Rogers, P.T; Coleman, M., *Medical Care in Down's Syndrome: A Preventive Medicine Approach,* Marcel Dekker, 1992.

68. Salmelin, R; Schnitzler, A; Schmitz, F; Jäncke, L; Witte, O.W; Freund, H.-J., 'Functional organization of the auditory cortex is different in stutterers and fluent speakers,' *NeuroReport,* Vol. 9, Issue 10, 13 July 1998, pp.2225-2229.

69. Seaman RL., 'Non-osseous sound transmission to the inner ear,' *Hearing Research,* 166, 2002, pp.214-215. Cited on: http://onderwijs1.amc.nl/medfysica/doc/Bone%20conduction.htm

70. Sekulowicz, M.G., 'The Role Of Early Diagnosis And Therapy Of ADHD,' Proceedings of the Tenth Biennial Conference of the International Association of Special Education, Hong Kong, June 2007.

71. Shambaugh G.E. Jr., 'The diagnosis and treatment of active cochlear otosclerosis,' *J. Laryngol Otol.,* Vol.85, 1971, pp.301-314. Cited 13th August 2009 on: http://www.dizziness-and-balance.com/disorders/hearing/otoscler.html

72. Shaywitz, S.E. and Shaywitz, 'The Neurobiology of Reading and Dyslexia,' *Focus on Basics,* National Center for the Study of Adult Learning and Literacy, Vol. 5, Issue A, August 2001.

73. Shealy, C. N., *Natural Progesterone Cream, Safe and Natural Hormone Replacement,* Keats, Lincolnwood, Illinois, 1999.

74. Sidlauskas, 'Language, the ideas of Director A. A. Tomatis as presented by A. E. Sidlauskas,' *Revue Internationale d'Audiopsychophonologie,* 1974.

75. *Sleep Mechanics,* Harvard Health Publications, October 1, 2007.

76. Snashall, S., 'Hearing Impairment and Down's Syndrome,' Cited on 7th Sept 2009: http://www.intellectualdisability.info/complex disability/P hearing ds.htm

77. Stehli, A. *The Sound of a Miracle: A Child's Triumph over Autism,* Doubleday, New York, 1991.

78. *The Mindd Handbook: An Integrative approach to treating ADHD, Allergies, Autism, Asthma and neuro-biological illness,* The MINDD Foundation, 2007. www.mindd.org

79. Thompson, B., 'Listening Disabilities: The Plight of Many,' in *Perspectives on Listening,* eds, Wolvyn, A; and Coakley, C. G., Ablex, New Jersey, 1993.

80. Tomatis, A. A., *The Ear and Language.* Moulin, Ontario, 1996.

81. Tomatis, A. A., *Vers l'Écoute Humaine,* Vols. 1 and 2. Les éditions ESF, Paris, 1974.

82. Tomatis, A.A., *The Conscious Ear,* Station Hill Press, New York, 1991.

83. Tremblay, K. L. 'Hearing Aids and the Brain: What's the Connection?' *The Hearing Journal,* Vol. 59, No. 8, August 2006, p.10.

84. 'Types of Hearing Loss. Dangerous Decibels: a public health partnership for the prevention of noise induced hearing loss,' Cited on 13th Sept 2009: http://www.dangerousdecibels.org/hearingloss.cfm

85. Van Jaarsveld, P.E; and Du Plessis, W.F., 'Audio-psycho-phonology at Potchefstroom: a review,' *South Africa Tydskr. Sielk (South African Journal of Psychology),* Vol. 18, No.4, 1988, pp.136-142.

86. Wakefield AJ, et al, 'Ileal-lymphoid-nodular hyperplasia, non-specific colitis, and

pervasive developmental disorder in children,' *Lancet*, 28;351(9103) Feb 1998, pp.637-641.

87. Weeks, Bradford S., 'The Therapeutic Effect of High Frequency Audition and its Role in Sacred Music;' in *About the Tomatis Method*, eds. Gilmor, Timothy M., Ph.D; Madaule, Paul, L.Ps; Thompson, Billie, Ph.D., The Listening Centre Press, Toronto, 1989. Cited on http://weeksmd.com/?p=714

88. http://en.wikipedia.org/wiki/Tensor_tympani

89. Whitwell, G. E., 'The Importance of Prenatal Sound and Music,' *The Journal of Prenatal & Perinatal Psychology and Health,* Cited on 7th Sept 2009 on: http://www.birthpsychology.com/lifebefore/sound1.html

90. Wenner, M., 'The Serious Need for Play,' *Scientific American Mind*, 39, Feb 2009.

91. Willott, J. 'Physiological Plasticity in the Auditory System and its Possible Relevance to Hearing Aid Use, Deprivation Effects, and Acclimatization,' *Ear and Hearing*, Vol. 17, Issue 3, June 1996, pp.66S-77S.

Index

Entries in **bold** refer to major references.
Entries in *italics* refer to books, videos, illustrations, tables or charts.

The Next Step

The great gift of Patricia and Rafaele Joudry's Sound Therapy is that it not only informs you about the harmful and healing effects of sound, it gives you an easy and efficient way of applying this knowledge to your own life. The self-help Sound Therapy program is simple to use and requires no time commitment, since the music is played at low volume during your normal daily activities.

Now that you are aware of the difference between harmful and healing sounds, you have the power of choice to take care of those marvellous instruments, your ears, and bathe them daily in the therapeutic high frequencies for which they were designed.

Sound Therapy listening programs

Our Sound Therapy self-help programs come as a convenient package with all the elements you need to conduct your listening at home.

These include:

- A course of progressively filtered Sound Therapy music
- A portable music player with the right specifications
- Suitable, light-weight, comfortable, high quality headphones
- A *Listeners Workbook* to guide you through the program
- Nutrition for the ears and brain.

The portable system offers you

- a very affordable price
- no fees for testing or supervision
- no need to travel for clinic treatment.

For details on the latest technology and current packages and pricing, or for any other questions you may have, contact one of our trained consultants who will be pleased to speak with you and advise you over the phone, or visit our website to learn more, or to find a consultant near you.

Contact details for Sound Therapy International

www.SoundTherapyInternational.com
email: info@SoundTherapyInternational.com
USA Phone 1800 323 9956
Australia Phone 1300 55 77 96

Other contact details available on website